INSTANT VORTEX

AIR FRYER RECIPES 2022

MANY TASTY RECIPES TO SURPRISE YOUR GUESTS

HENRY KING

Table of Contents

Curried Orange Honey Chicken

Prep time: 10 minutes | Cook time: 16 to 19 minutes | Serves 4

¾ pound (340 g) boneless, skinless chicken thighs, cut into 1-inch pieces

1 yellow bell pepper, cut into 1½-inch pieces

1 small red onion, sliced

Olive oil for misting

¼ cup chicken stock

2 tablespoons honey

¼ cup orange juice

1 tablespoon cornstarch

2 to 3 teaspoons curry powder

1. Set the temperature of the air fryer oven to 370ºF (188ºC). Press Start to begin preheating.
2. Put the chicken thighs, pepper, and red onion in the air fryer oven perforated pan and mist with olive oil.
3. Roast for 12 to 14 minutes or until the chicken is cooked to 165ºF (74ºC), shaking the perforated pan halfway through cooking time.
4. Remove the chicken and vegetables from the air fryer oven perforated pan and set aside.

5. In a metal bowl, combine the stock, honey, orange juice, cornstarch, and curry powder, and mix well. Add the chicken and vegetables, stir, and put the bowl in the oven.

6. Roast for 2 minutes. Remove and stir, then roast for 2 to 3 minutes or until the sauce is thickened and bubbly.

7. Serve warm.

Dill Chicken Strips

Prep time: 15 minutes | Cook time: 10 minutes | Serves 4

2 whole boneless, skinless chicken breasts, halved lengthwise

1 cup Italian dressing

3 cups finely crushed potato chips

1 tablespoon dried dill weed

1 tablespoon garlic powder

1 large egg, beaten

Cooking spray

1. In a large resealable bag, combine the chicken and Italian dressing. Seal the bag and refrigerate to marinate at least 1 hour.

2. In a shallow dish, stir together the potato chips, dill, and garlic powder. Place the beaten egg in a second shallow dish.

3. Remove the chicken from the marinade. Roll the chicken pieces in the egg and the potato chip mixture, coating thoroughly.

4. Set the temperature of the air fryer oven to 325ºF (163ºC). Press Start to begin preheating. Line the air fryer oven perforated pan with parchment paper.

5. Place the coated chicken on the parchment and spritz with cooking spray.

6. Bake for 5 minutes. Flip the chicken, spritz with cooking spray, and bake for 5 minutes more until the outsides are crispy and the insides are no longer pink. Serve immediately.

Easy Asian Turkey Meatballs

Prep time: 10 minutes | Cook time: 11 to 14 minutes | Serves 4

2 tablespoons peanut oil, divided

1 small onion, minced

¼ cup water chestnuts, finely chopped

½ teaspoon ground ginger

2 tablespoons low-sodium soy sauce

¼ cup panko bread crumbs

1 egg, beaten

1 pound (454 g) ground turkey

1. Set the temperature of the air fryer oven to 400ºF (204ºC). Press Start to begin preheating.

2. In a round metal pan, combine 1 tablespoon of peanut oil and onion. Air fry for 1 to 2 minutes or until crisp and tender. Transfer the onion to a medium bowl.

3. Add the water chestnuts, ground ginger, soy sauce, and bread crumbs to the onion and mix well. Add egg and stir well. Mix in the ground turkey until combined.

4. Form the mixture into 1-inch meatballs. Drizzle the remaining 1 tablespoon of oil over the meatballs.

5. Bake the meatballs in the pan in batches for 10 to 12 minutes or until they are 165ºF (74ºC) on a meat thermometer. Rest for 5 minutes before serving.

Easy Tandoori Chicken

Prep time: 5 minutes | Cook time: 18 to 23 minutes | Serves 4

$^2/_3$ cup plain low-fat yogurt

2 tablespoons freshly squeezed lemon juice

2 teaspoons curry powder

½ teaspoon ground cinnamon

2 garlic cloves, minced

2 teaspoons olive oil

4 (5-ounce / 142-g) low-sodium boneless, skinless chicken breasts

1. In a medium bowl, whisk the yogurt, lemon juice, curry powder, cinnamon, garlic, and olive oil.

2. With a sharp knife, cut thin slashes into the chicken. Add it to the yogurt mixture and turn to coat. Let stand for 10 minutes at room temperature. You can also prepare this ahead of time and marinate the chicken in the refrigerator for up to 24 hours.

3. Set the temperature of the air fryer oven to 360ºF (182ºC). Press Start to begin preheating.

4. Remove the chicken from the marinade and shake off any excess liquid. Discard any remaining marinade.

5. Roast the chicken for 10 minutes. With tongs, carefully turn each piece. Roast for 8 to 13 minutes more, or until the chicken reaches an internal temperature of 165ºF (74ºC) on a meat thermometer. Serve immediately.

Crispy Chicken Strips

Prep time: 15 minutes | Cook time: 20 minutes | Serves 4

1 tablespoon olive oil

1 pound (454 g) boneless, skinless chicken tenderloins

1 teaspoon salt

½ teaspoon freshly ground black pepper

½ teaspoon paprika

½ teaspoon garlic powder

½ cup whole-wheat seasoned bread crumbs

1 teaspoon dried parsley

Cooking spray

1. Set the temperature of the air fryer oven to 370ºF (188ºC). Press Start to begin preheating. Spray the air fryer oven perforated pan lightly with cooking spray.

2. In a medium bowl, toss the chicken with the salt, pepper, paprika, and garlic powder until evenly coated.

3. Add the olive oil and toss to coat the chicken evenly.

4. In a separate, shallow bowl, mix together the bread crumbs and parsley.

5. Coat each piece of chicken evenly in the bread crumb mixture.

6. Place the chicken in the air fryer oven perforated pan in a single layer and spray it lightly with cooking spray. You may need to cook them in batches.

7. Air fry for 10 minutes. Flip the chicken over, lightly spray it with cooking spray, and air fry for an additional 8 to 10 minutes, until golden brown. Serve.

Fajita Chicken Strips

Prep time: 10 minutes | Cook time: 15 minutes | Serves 4

1 pound (454 g) boneless, skinless chicken tenderloins, cut into strips

3 bell peppers, any color, cut into chunks

1 onion, cut into chunks

1 tablespoon olive oil, plus more for spraying

1 tablespoon fajita seasoning mix

Cooking spray

1. Set the temperature of the air fryer oven to 370ºF (188ºC). Press Start to begin preheating.

2. In a large bowl, mix together the chicken, bell peppers, onion, olive oil, and fajita seasoning mix until completely coated.

3. Spray the air fryer oven perforated pan lightly with cooking spray.

4. Place the chicken and vegetables in the air fryer oven perforated pan and lightly spray with cooking spray.

5. Air fry for 7 minutes. Shake the perforated pan and air fry for an additional 5 to 8 minutes, until the chicken is cooked through and the veggies are starting to char.

6. Serve warm.

Fried Buffalo Chicken Taquitos

Prep time: 15 minutes | Cook time: 5 to 10 minutes | Serves 6

8 ounces (227 g) fat-free cream cheese, softened

⅛ cup Buffalo sauce

2 cups shredded cooked chicken

12 (7-inch) low-carb flour tortillas

Cooking spray

1. Set the temperature of the air fryer oven to 360ºF (182ºC). Press Start to begin preheating. Spray the air fryer oven perforated pan lightly with cooking spray.

2. In a large bowl, mix together the cream cheese and Buffalo sauce until well combined. Add the chicken and stir until combined.

3. Place the tortillas on a clean workspace. Spoon 2 to 3 tablespoons of the chicken mixture in a thin line down the center of each tortilla. Roll up the tortillas.

4. Place the tortillas in the air fryer oven perforated pan, seam-side down. Spray each tortilla lightly with cooking spray. You may need to cook the taquitos in batches.

5. Air fry until golden brown, 5 to 10 minutes. Serve hot.

Garlic Soy Chicken Thighs

Prep time: 10 minutes | Cook time: 30 minutes | Serves 1 to 2

2 tablespoons chicken stock

2 tablespoons reduced-sodium soy sauce

1½ tablespoons sugar

4 garlic cloves, smashed and peeled

2 large scallions, cut into 2- to 3-inch batons, plus more, thinly sliced, for garnish

2 bone-in, skin-on chicken thighs (7 to 8 ounces / 198 to 227 g each)

1. Set the temperature of the air fryer oven to 375ºF (191ºC). Press Start to begin preheating.

2. In a metal cake pan, combine the chicken stock, soy sauce, and sugar and stir until the sugar dissolves. Add the garlic cloves, scallions, and chicken thighs, turning the thighs to coat them in the marinade, then resting them skin-side up. Place the pan in the air fryer oven and bake, flipping the thighs every 5 minutes after the first 10 minutes, until the chicken is cooked through and the marinade is reduced to a sticky glaze over the chicken, about 30 minutes.

3. Remove the pan from the air fryer oven and serve the chicken thighs warm, with any remaining glaze spooned over top and sprinkled with more sliced scallions.

Ginger Chicken Thighs

Prep time: 10 minutes | Cook time: 10 minutes | Serves 4

¼ cup julienned peeled fresh ginger

2 tablespoons vegetable oil

1 tablespoon honey

1 tablespoon soy sauce

1 tablespoon ketchup

1 teaspoon garam masala

1 teaspoon ground turmeric

¼ teaspoon kosher salt

½ teaspoon cayenne pepper

Vegetable oil spray

1 pound (454 g) boneless, skinless chicken thighs, cut crosswise into thirds

¼ cup chopped fresh cilantro, for garnish

1. In a small bowl, combine the ginger, oil, honey, soy sauce, ketchup, garam masala, turmeric, salt, and cayenne. Whisk until well combined. Place the chicken in a resealable plastic bag and pour the marinade over. Seal the bag and massage to cover all of the chicken with the marinade. Marinate at room temperature for 30 minutes or in the refrigerator for up to 24 hours.

2. Set the temperature of the air fryer oven to 350ºF (177ºC). Press Start to begin preheating.

3. Spray the air fryer oven perforated pan with vegetable oil spray and add the chicken and as much of the marinade and julienned ginger as possible. Bake for 10 minutes. Use a meat thermometer to ensure the chicken has reached an internal temperature of 165ºF (74ºC).

4. To serve, garnish with cilantro.

Glazed Chicken Drumsticks

Prep time: 5 minutes | Cook time: 20 minutes | Serves 2

4 chicken drumsticks

3 tablespoons soy sauce

2 tablespoons brown sugar

1 teaspoon minced garlic

1 teaspoon minced fresh ginger

1 teaspoon toasted sesame oil

½ teaspoon red pepper flakes

½ teaspoon kosher salt

½ teaspoon black pepper

1. Set the temperature of the air fryer oven to 400ºF (204ºC). Press Start to begin preheating.

2. Line a round baking pan with aluminum foil. (If you don't do this, you'll either end up scrubbing forever or throwing out the pan.) Arrange the drumsticks in the prepared pan.

3. In a medium bowl, stir together the soy sauce, brown sugar, garlic, ginger, sesame oil, red pepper flakes, salt, and black pepper. Pour the sauce over the drumsticks and toss to coat.

4. Place the pan in the air fryer oven. Air fry for 20 minutes, turning the drumsticks halfway through the cooking time. Use a meat thermometer to ensure the chicken has reached an internal temperature of 165ºF (74ºC). Serve immediately.

Hawaiian Tropical Chicken

Prep time: 10 minutes | Cook time: 15 minutes | Serves 4

4 boneless, skinless chicken thighs (about 1½ pounds / 680 g)

1 (8-ounce / 227-g) can pineapple chunks in juice, drained, ¼ cup juice reserved

¼ cup soy sauce

¼ cup sugar

2 tablespoons ketchup

1 tablespoon minced fresh ginger

1 tablespoon minced garlic

¼ cup chopped scallions

1. Use a fork to pierce the chicken all over to allow the marinade to penetrate better. Place the chicken in a large bowl or large resealable plastic bag.

2. Set the drained pineapple chunks aside. In a small microwave-safe bowl, combine the pineapple juice, soy sauce, sugar, ketchup, ginger, and garlic. Pour half the sauce over the chicken; toss to coat. Reserve the remaining sauce. Marinate the chicken at room temperature for 30 minutes, or cover and refrigerate for up to 24 hours.

3. Set the temperature of the air fryer oven to 350ºF (177ºC). Press Start to begin preheating.

4. Place the chicken in the air fryer oven perforated pan, discarding marinade. Bake for 15 minutes, turning halfway through the cooking time.

5. Meanwhile, microwave the reserved sauce on high for 45 to 60 seconds, stirring every 15 seconds, until the sauce has the consistency of a thick glaze.

6. At the end of the cooking time, use a meat thermometer to ensure the chicken has reached an internal temperature of 165ºF (74ºC).

7. Transfer the chicken to a serving platter. Pour the sauce over the chicken. Garnish with the pineapple chunks and scallions before serving.

Herb-Buttermilk Chicken Breast

Prep time: 5 minutes | Cook time: 40 minutes | Serves 2

1 large bone-in, skin-on chicken breast

1 cup buttermilk

1½ teaspoons dried parsley

1½ teaspoons dried chives

¾ teaspoon kosher salt

½ teaspoon dried dill

½ teaspoon onion powder

¼ teaspoon garlic powder

¼ teaspoon dried tarragon

Cooking spray

1. Place the chicken breast in a bowl and pour over the buttermilk, turning the chicken in it to make sure it's completely covered. Let the chicken stand at room temperature for at least 20 minutes or in the refrigerator for up to 4 hours.

2. Meanwhile, in a bowl, stir together the parsley, chives, salt, dill, onion powder, garlic powder, and tarragon.

3. Set the temperature of the air fryer oven to 300ºF (149ºC). Press Start to begin preheating.

4. Remove the chicken from the buttermilk, letting the excess drip off, then place the chicken skin-side up directly in the air fryer oven. Sprinkle the seasoning mix all over the top of the chicken breast, then let stand until the herb mix soaks into the buttermilk, at least 5 minutes.

5. Spray the top of the chicken with cooking spray. Bake for 10 minutes, then increase the temperature to 350ºF (177ºC) and bake until an instant-read thermometer inserted into the thickest part of the breast reads 160ºF (71ºC) and the chicken is deep golden brown, 30 to 35 minutes.

6. Transfer the chicken breast to a cutting board, let rest for 10 minutes, then cut the meat off the bone and cut into thick slices for serving.

Herbed Turkey Breast

Prep time: 20 minutes | Cook time: 45 minutes | Serves 6

1 tablespoon olive oil

Cooking spray

2 garlic cloves, minced

2 teaspoons Dijon mustard

1½ teaspoons rosemary

1½ teaspoons sage

1½ teaspoons thyme

1 teaspoon salt

½ teaspoon freshly ground black pepper

3 pounds (1.4 kg) turkey breast, thawed if frozen

1. Set the temperature of the air fryer oven to 370ºF (188ºC). Press Start to begin preheating. Spray the air fryer oven perforated pan lightly with cooking spray.

2. In a small bowl, mix together the garlic, olive oil, Dijon mustard, rosemary, sage, thyme, salt, and pepper to make a paste. Smear the paste all over the turkey breast.

3. Place the turkey breast in the air fryer oven perforated pan. Air fry for 20 minutes. Flip turkey breast over and baste it with any drippings that have collected in the

bottom drawer of the air fryer oven. Air fry until the internal temperature of the meat reaches at least 170ºF (77ºC), 20 more minutes.

4. If desired, increase the temperature to 400ºF (204ºC), flip the turkey breast over one last time, and air fry for 5 minutes to get a crispy exterior.

5. Let the turkey rest for 10 minutes before slicing and serving.

Honey Rosemary Chicken

Prep time: 10 minutes | Cook time: 20 minutes | Serves 4

¼ cup balsamic vinegar

¼ cup honey

2 tablespoons olive oil

1 tablespoon dried rosemary leaves

1 teaspoon salt

½ teaspoon freshly ground black pepper

2 whole boneless, skinless chicken breasts (about 1 pound / 454 g each), halved

Cooking spray

1. In a large resealable bag, combine the vinegar, honey, olive oil, rosemary, salt, and pepper. Add the chicken pieces, seal the bag, and refrigerate to marinate for at least 2 hours.

2. Set the temperature of the air fryer oven to 325ºF (163ºC). Press Start to begin preheating. Line the air fryer oven perforated pan with parchment paper.

3. Remove the chicken from the marinade and place it on the parchment. Spritz with cooking spray.

4. Bake for 10 minutes. Flip the chicken, spritz with cooking spray, and bake for 10 minutes more until the internal temperature reaches 165ºF (74ºC) and the chicken is no longer pink inside. Let sit for 5 minutes before serving.

Israeli Chicken Schnitzel

Prep time: 5 minutes | Cook time: 10 minutes | Serves 4

2 large boneless, skinless chicken breasts, each weighing about 1 pound (454 g)

1 cup all-purpose flour

2 teaspoons garlic powder

2 teaspoons kosher salt

1 teaspoon black pepper

1 teaspoon paprika

2 eggs beaten with 2 tablespoons water

2 cups panko bread crumbs

Vegetable oil spray

Lemon juice, for serving

1. Set the temperature of the air fryer oven to 375ºF (191ºC). Press Start to begin preheating.

2. Place 1 chicken breast between 2 pieces of plastic wrap. Use a mallet or a rolling pin to pound the chicken until it is ¼ inch thick. Set aside. Repeat with the second breast. Whisk together the flour, garlic powder, salt, pepper, and paprika on a large plate. Place the panko in a separate shallow bowl or pie plate.

3. Dredge 1 chicken breast in the flour, shaking off any excess, then dip it in the egg mixture. Dredge the chicken breast in the panko, making sure to coat it completely. Shake off any excess panko. Place the battered chicken breast on a plate. Repeat with the second chicken breast.

4. Spray the air fryer oven perforated pan with oil spray. Place 1 of the battered chicken breasts in the perforated pan and spray the top with oil spray. Air fry until the top is browned, about 5 minutes. Flip the chicken and spray the second side with oil spray. Air fry until the second side is browned and crispy and the internal temperature reaches 165ºF (74ºC). Remove the first chicken breast from the air fryer oven and repeat with the second chicken breast.

5. Serve hot with lemon juice.

Jerk Chicken Leg Quarters

Prep time: 8 minutes | Cook time: 27 minutes | Serves 2

1 tablespoon packed brown sugar

1 teaspoon ground allspice

1 teaspoon pepper

1 teaspoon garlic powder

¾ teaspoon dry mustard

¾ teaspoon dried thyme

½ teaspoon salt

¼ teaspoon cayenne pepper

2 (10-ounce / 284-g) chicken leg quarters, trimmed

1 teaspoon vegetable oil

1 scallion, green part only, sliced thin

Lime wedges

1. Set the temperature of the air fryer oven to 400ºF (204ºC). Press Start to begin preheating.

2. Combine sugar, allspice, pepper, garlic powder, mustard, thyme, salt, and cayenne in a bowl. Pat chicken dry with paper towels. Using metal skewer, poke 10 to 15 holes in skin of each chicken leg. Rub with oil and sprinkle evenly with spice mixture.

3. Arrange chicken skin-side up in the air fryer oven perforated pan, spaced evenly apart. Air fry until chicken is well browned and crisp, 27 to 30 minutes, rotating chicken halfway through cooking (do not flip).

4. Transfer chicken to plate, tent loosely with aluminum foil, and let rest for 5 minutes. Sprinkle with scallion. Serve with lime wedges.

Lemon Chicken and Spinach Salad

Prep time: 10 minutes | Cook time: 16 to 20 minutes | Serves 4

3 (5-ounce / 142-g) low-sodium boneless, skinless chicken breasts, cut into 1-inch cubes

5 teaspoons olive oil

½ teaspoon dried thyme

1 medium red onion, sliced

1 red bell pepper, sliced

1 small zucchini, cut into strips

3 tablespoons freshly squeezed lemon juice

6 cups fresh baby spinach

1. Set the temperature of the air fryer oven to 400ºF (204ºC). Press Start to begin preheating.

2. In a large bowl, mix the chicken with the olive oil and thyme. Toss to coat. Transfer to a medium metal bowl and roast for 8 minutes in the air fryer oven.

3. Add the red onion, red bell pepper, and zucchini. Roast for 8 to 12 minutes more, stirring once during cooking, or until the chicken reaches an internal temperature of 165ºF (74ºC) on a meat thermometer.

4. Remove the bowl from the air fryer oven and stir in the lemon juice.

5. Put the spinach in a serving bowl and top with the chicken mixture. Toss to combine and serve immediately.

Lemon Garlic Chicken

Prep time: 10 minutes | Cook time: 16 to 19 minutes | Serves 4

4 (5-ounce / 142-g) low-sodium boneless, skinless chicken breasts, cut into 4-by-½-inch strips

2 teaspoons olive oil

2 tablespoons cornstarch

3 garlic cloves, minced

½ cup low-sodium chicken broth

¼ cup freshly squeezed lemon juice

1 tablespoon honey

½ teaspoon dried thyme

1. Set the temperature of the air fryer oven to 400ºF (204ºC). Press Start to begin preheating.

2. In a large bowl, mix the chicken and olive oil. Sprinkle with the cornstarch. Toss to coat.

3. Add the garlic and transfer to a metal pan. Bake in the air fryer oven for 10 minutes, stirring once during cooking.

4. Add the chicken broth, lemon juice, honey, and thyme to the chicken mixture. Bake for 6 to 9 minutes more, or until the sauce is slightly thickened and the chicken reaches an internal temperature of 165ºF (74ºC) on a meat thermometer. Serve over hot cooked brown rice, if desired.

Lemon Parmesan Chicken

Prep time: 10 minutes | Cook time: 20 minutes | Serves 4

1 egg

2 tablespoons lemon juice

2 teaspoons minced garlic

½ teaspoon salt

½ teaspoon freshly ground black pepper

4 boneless, skinless chicken breasts, thin cut

Cooking spray

½ cup whole-wheat bread crumbs

¼ cup grated Parmesan cheese

1. In a medium bowl, whisk together the egg, lemon juice, garlic, salt, and pepper. Add the chicken breasts, cover, and refrigerate for up to 1 hour.

2. In a shallow bowl, combine the bread crumbs and Parmesan cheese.

3. Set the temperature of the air fryer oven to 360ºF (182ºC). Press Start to begin preheating. Spray the air fryer oven perforated pan lightly with cooking spray.

4. Remove the chicken breasts from the egg mixture, then dredge them in the bread crumb mixture, and place in the air fryer oven perforated pan in a single layer. Lightly spray the chicken breasts with cooking spray. You may need to cook the chicken in batches.

5. Air fry for 8 minutes. Flip the chicken over, lightly spray with cooking spray, and air fry until the chicken reaches an internal temperature of 165ºF (74ºC), for an additional 7 to 12 minutes.

6. Serve warm.

Mayonnaise-Mustard Chicken

Prep time: 10 minutes | Cook time: 15 minutes | Serves 4

6 tablespoons mayonnaise

2 tablespoons coarse-ground mustard

2 teaspoons honey (optional)

2 teaspoons curry powder

1 teaspoon kosher salt

1 teaspoon cayenne pepper

1 pound (454 g) chicken tenders

1. Set the temperature of the air fryer oven to 350ºF (177ºC). Press Start to begin preheating.

2. In a large bowl, whisk together the mayonnaise, mustard, honey (if using), curry powder, salt, and cayenne. Transfer half of the mixture to a serving bowl to serve as a dipping sauce. Add the chicken tenders to the large bowl and toss until well coated.

3. Place the tenders in the air fryer oven perforated pan and bake for 15 minutes. Use a meat thermometer to ensure the chicken has reached an internal temperature of 165ºF (74ºC).

4. Serve the chicken with the dipping sauce.

Merguez Meatballs

Prep time: 10 minutes | Cook time: 10 minutes | Serves 4

1 pound (454 g) ground chicken

2 garlic cloves, finely minced

1 tablespoon sweet Hungarian paprika

1 teaspoon kosher salt

1 teaspoon sugar

1 teaspoon ground cumin

½ teaspoon black pepper

½ teaspoon ground fennel

½ teaspoon ground coriander

½ teaspoon cayenne pepper

¼ teaspoon ground allspice

1. In a large bowl, gently mix the chicken, garlic, paprika, salt, sugar, cumin, black pepper, fennel, coriander, cayenne, and allspice until all the ingredients are incorporated. Let stand for 30 minutes at room temperature, or cover and refrigerate for up to 24 hours.

2. Set the temperature of the air fryer oven to 400ºF (204ºC). Press Start to begin preheating.

3. Form the mixture into 16 meatballs. Arrange them in a single layer in the air fryer oven perforated pan. Air fry for 10 minutes, turning the meatballs halfway through the cooking time. Use a meat thermometer to ensure the meatballs have reached an internal temperature of 165ºF (74ºC).

4. Serve warm.

Mini Turkey Meatloaves with Carrot

Prep time: 6 minutes | Cook time: 20 to 24 minutes | Serves 4

$^1/_3$ cup minced onion

¼ cup grated carrot

2 garlic cloves, minced

2 tablespoons ground almonds

2 teaspoons olive oil

1 teaspoon dried marjoram

1 egg white

¾ pound (340 g) ground turkey breast

1. Set the temperature of the air fryer oven to 400ºF (204ºC). Press Start to begin preheating.

2. In a medium bowl, stir together the onion, carrot, garlic, almonds, olive oil, marjoram, and egg white.

3. Add the ground turkey. With the hands, gently but thoroughly mix until combined.

4. Double 16 foil muffin cup liners to make 8 cups. Divide the turkey mixture evenly among the liners.

5. Bake for 20 to 24 minutes, or until the meatloaves reach an internal temperature of 165ºF (74ºC) on a meat thermometer. Serve immediately.

Nutty Chicken Tenders

Prep time: 5 minutes | Cook time: 12 minutes | Serves 4

1 pound (454 g) chicken tenders

1 teaspoon kosher salt

1 teaspoon black pepper

½ teaspoon smoked paprika

¼ cup coarse mustard

2 tablespoons honey

1 cup finely crushed pecans

1. Set the temperature of the air fryer oven to 350ºF (177ºC). Press Start to begin preheating.

2. Place the chicken in a large bowl. Sprinkle with the salt, pepper, and paprika. Toss until the chicken is coated with the spices. Add the mustard and honey and toss until the chicken is coated.

3. Place the pecans on a plate. Working with one piece of chicken at a time, roll the chicken in the pecans until both sides are coated. Lightly brush off any loose pecans. Place the chicken in the air fryer oven perforated pan.

4. Bake for 12 minutes, or until the chicken is cooked through and the pecans are golden brown.

5. Serve warm.

Orange and Honey Glazed Duck with Apples

Prep time: 5 minutes | Cook time: 15 minutes | Serves 2 to 3

1 pound (454 g) duck breasts (2 to 3 breasts)

Kosher salt and pepper, to taste

Juice and zest of 1 orange

¼ cup honey

2 sprigs thyme, plus more for garnish

2 firm tart apples, such as Fuji

1. Set the temperature of the air fryer oven to 400ºF (204ºC). Press Start to begin preheating.

2. Pat the duck breasts dry and, using a sharp knife, make 3 to 4 shallow, diagonal slashes in the skin. Turn the breasts and score the skin on the diagonal in the opposite direction to create a cross-hatch pattern. Season well with salt and pepper.

3. Place the duck breasts skin-side up in the air fryer oven perforated pan. Roast for 8 minutes, then flip and roast for 4 more minutes on the second side.

4. While the duck is cooking, prepare the sauce. Combine the orange juice and zest, honey, and thyme in a small saucepan. Bring to a boil, stirring to dissolve the honey, then reduce the heat and simmer until thickened. Core

the apples and cut into quarters. Cut each quarter into 3 or 4 slices depending on the size.

5. After the duck has cooked on both sides, turn it and brush the skin with the orange-honey glaze. Roast for 1 more minute. Remove the duck breasts to a cutting board and allow to rest.

6. Toss the apple slices with the remaining orange-honey sauce in a medium bowl. Arrange the apples in a single layer in the air fryer oven perforated pan. Air fry for 10 minutes while the duck breast rests. Slice the duck breasts on the bias and divide them and the apples among 2 or 3 plates.

7. Serve warm, garnished with additional thyme.

Paprika Indian Fennel Chicken

Prep time: 10 minutes | Cook time: 15 minutes | Serves 4

1 pound (454 g) boneless, skinless chicken thighs, cut crosswise into thirds

1 yellow onion, cut into 1½-inch-thick slices

1 tablespoon coconut oil, melted

2 teaspoons minced fresh ginger

2 teaspoons minced garlic

1 teaspoon smoked paprika

1 teaspoon ground fennel

1 teaspoon garam masala

1 teaspoon ground turmeric

1 teaspoon kosher salt

½ to 1 teaspoon cayenne pepper

Vegetable oil spray

2 teaspoons fresh lemon juice

¼ cup chopped fresh cilantro or parsley

1. Use a fork to pierce the chicken all over to allow the marinade to penetrate better.

2. In a large bowl, combine the onion, coconut oil, ginger, garlic, paprika, fennel, garam masala, turmeric, salt,

and cayenne. Add the chicken, toss to combine, and marinate at room temperature for 30 minutes, or cover and refrigerate for up to 24 hours.

3. Set the temperature of the air fryer oven to 350ºF (177ºC). Press Start to begin preheating.

4. Place the chicken and onion in the air fryer oven perforated pan. (Discard remaining marinade.) Spray with some vegetable oil spray. Air fry for 15 minutes. Halfway through the cooking time, remove the perforated pan, spray the chicken and onion with more vegetable oil spray, and toss gently to coat. At the end of the cooking time, use a meat thermometer to ensure the chicken has reached an internal temperature of 165ºF (74ºC).

5. Transfer the chicken and onion to a serving platter. Sprinkle with the lemon juice and cilantro and serve.

Parmesan Chicken Wings

Prep time: 15 minutes | Cook time: 16 to 18 minutes | Serves 4

1¼ cups grated Parmesan cheese

1 tablespoon garlic powder

1 teaspoon salt

½ teaspoon freshly ground black pepper

¾ cup all-purpose flour

1 large egg, beaten

12 chicken wings (about 1 pound / 454 g)

Cooking spray

1. Set the temperature of the air fryer oven to 390ºF (199ºC). Press Start to begin preheating. Line the air fryer oven perforated pan with parchment paper.

2. In a shallow bowl, whisk the Parmesan cheese, garlic powder, salt, and pepper until blended. Place the flour in a second shallow bowl and the beaten egg in a third shallow bowl.

3. One at a time, dip the chicken wings into the flour, the beaten egg, and the Parmesan cheese mixture, coating thoroughly.

4. Place the chicken wings on the parchment and spritz with cooking spray.

5. Air fry for 8 minutes. Flip the chicken, spritz it with cooking spray, and air fry for 8 to 10 minutes more until the internal temperature reaches 165ºF (74ºC) and the insides are no longer pink. Let sit for 5 minutes before serving.

Pecan-Crusted Turkey Cutlets

Prep time: 10 minutes | Cook time: 10 to 12 minutes | Serves 4

¾ cup panko bread crumbs

¼ teaspoon salt

¼ teaspoon pepper

¼ teaspoon dry mustard

¼ teaspoon poultry seasoning

½ cup pecans

¼ cup cornstarch

1 egg, beaten

1 pound (454 g) turkey cutlets, ½-inch thick

Salt and pepper, to taste

Cooking spray

1. Set the temperature of the air fryer oven to 360ºF (182ºC). Press Start to begin preheating.

2. Place the panko crumbs, salt, pepper, mustard, and poultry seasoning in a food processor. Process until crumbs are finely crushed. Add pecans and process just until nuts are finely chopped.

3. Place cornstarch in a shallow dish and beaten egg in another. Transfer coating mixture from food processor into a third shallow dish.

4. Sprinkle turkey cutlets with salt and pepper to taste.

5. Dip cutlets in cornstarch and shake off excess, then dip in beaten egg and finally roll in crumbs, pressing to coat well. Spray both sides with cooking spray.

6. Place 2 cutlets in air fryer oven perforated pan in a single layer and air fry for 10 to 12 minutes. Repeat with the remaining cutlets.

7. Serve warm.

Piri-Piri Chicken Thighs

Prep time: 5 minutes | Cook time: 25 minutes | Serves 4

¼ cup piri-piri sauce

1 tablespoon freshly squeezed lemon juice

2 tablespoons brown sugar, divided

2 cloves garlic, minced

1 tablespoon extra-virgin olive oil

4 bone-in, skin-on chicken thighs, each weighing approximately 7 to 8 ounces (198 to 227 g)

½ teaspoon cornstarch

1. To make the marinade, whisk together the piri-piri sauce, lemon juice, 1 tablespoon of brown sugar, and the garlic in a small bowl. While whisking, slowly pour in the oil in a steady stream and continue to whisk until emulsified. Using a skewer, poke holes in the chicken thighs and place them in a small glass dish. Pour the marinade over the chicken and turn the thighs to coat them with the sauce. Cover the dish and refrigerate for at least 15 minutes and up to 1 hour.

2. Set the temperature of the air fryer oven to 375ºF (191ºC). Press Start to begin preheating. Remove the chicken thighs from the dish, reserving the marinade, and place them skin-side down in the air fryer oven

perforated pan. Air fry until the internal temperature reaches 165ºF (74ºC), 15 to 20 minutes.

3. Meanwhile, whisk the remaining brown sugar and the cornstarch into the marinade and microwave it on high power for 1 minute until it is bubbling and thickened to a glaze.

4. Once the chicken is cooked, turn the thighs over and brush them with the glaze. Air fry for a few additional minutes until the glaze browns and begins to char in spots.

5. Remove the chicken to a platter and serve with additional piri-piri sauce, if desired.

Potato Cheese Crusted Chicken

Prep time: 15 minutes | Cook time: 22 to 25 minutes | Serves 4

¼ cup buttermilk

1 large egg, beaten

1 cup instant potato flakes

¼ cup grated Parmesan cheese

1 teaspoon salt

½ teaspoon freshly ground black pepper

2 whole boneless, skinless chicken breasts (about 1 pound / 454 g each), halved

Cooking spray

1. Set the temperature of the air fryer oven to 325ºF (163ºC). Press Start to begin preheating. Line the air fryer oven perforated pan with parchment paper.

2. In a shallow bowl, whisk the buttermilk and egg until blended. In another shallow bowl, stir together the potato flakes, cheese, salt, and pepper.

3. One at a time, dip the chicken pieces in the buttermilk mixture and the potato flake mixture, coating thoroughly.

4. Place the coated chicken on the parchment and spritz with cooking spray.

5. Bake for 15 minutes. Flip the chicken, spritz with cooking spray, and bake for 7 to 10 minutes more until the outside is crispy and the inside is no longer pink. Serve immediately.

Roasted Cajun Turkey

Prep time: 10 minutes | Cook time: 30 minutes | Serves 4

2 pounds (907 g) turkey thighs, skinless and boneless

1 red onion, sliced

2 bell peppers, sliced

1 habanero pepper, minced

1 carrot, sliced

1 tablespoon Cajun seasoning mix

1 tablespoon fish sauce

2 cups chicken broth

Nonstick cooking spray

1. Set the temperature of the air fryer oven to 360ºF (182ºC). Press Start to begin preheating.

2. Spritz the bottom and sides of a baking dish with nonstick cooking spray.

3. Arrange the turkey thighs in the baking dish. Add the onion, peppers, and carrot. Sprinkle with Cajun seasoning. Add the fish sauce and chicken broth.

4. Roast in the preheated air fryer oven for 30 minutes until cooked through. Serve warm.

Roasted Chicken and Vegetable Salad

Prep time: 10 minutes | Cook time: 10 to 13 minutes | Serves 4

3 (4-ounce / 113-g) low-sodium boneless, skinless chicken breasts, cut into 1-inch cubes

1 small red onion, sliced

1 red bell pepper, sliced

1 cup green beans, cut into 1-inch pieces

2 tablespoons low-fat ranch salad dressing

2 tablespoons freshly squeezed lemon juice

½ teaspoon dried basil

4 cups mixed lettuce

1. Set the temperature of the air fryer oven to 400ºF (204ºC). Press Start to begin preheating.

2. In the air fryer oven perforated pan, roast the chicken, red onion, red bell pepper, and green beans for 10 to 13 minutes, or until the chicken reaches an internal temperature of 165ºF (74ºC) on a meat thermometer, tossing the food in the perforated pan once during cooking.

3. While the chicken cooks, in a serving bowl, mix the ranch dressing, lemon juice, and basil.

4. Transfer the chicken and vegetables to a serving bowl and toss with the dressing to coat. Serve immediately on lettuce leaves.

Roasted Chicken Tenders with Veggies

Prep time: 10 minutes | Cook time: 18 to 20 minutes | Serves 4

1 pound (454 g) chicken tenders

1 tablespoon honey

Pinch salt

Freshly ground black pepper, to taste

½ cup soft fresh bread crumbs

½ teaspoon dried thyme

1 tablespoon olive oil

2 carrots, sliced

12 small red potatoes

1. Set the temperature of the air fryer oven to 380ºF (193ºC). Press Start to begin preheating.

2. In a medium bowl, toss the chicken tenders with the honey, salt, and pepper.

3. In a shallow bowl, combine the bread crumbs, thyme, and olive oil, and mix.

4. Coat the tenders in the bread crumbs, pressing firmly onto the meat.

5. Place the carrots and potatoes in the air fryer oven perforated pan and top with the chicken tenders.

6. Roast for 18 to 20 minutes or until the chicken is cooked to 165ºF (74ºC) and the vegetables are tender, shaking the perforated pan halfway during the cooking time.

7. Serve warm.

Roasted Chicken with Garlic

Prep time: 5 minutes | Cook time: 25 minutes | Serves 4

4 (5-ounce / 142-g) low-sodium bone-in skinless chicken breasts

1 tablespoon olive oil

1 tablespoon freshly squeezed lemon juice

3 tablespoons cornstarch

1 teaspoon dried basil leaves

⅛ teaspoon freshly ground black pepper

20 garlic cloves, unpeeled

1. Set the temperature of the air fryer oven to 370ºF (188ºC). Press Start to begin preheating.

2. Rub the chicken with the olive oil and lemon juice on both sides and sprinkle with the cornstarch, basil, and pepper.

3. Place the seasoned chicken in the air fryer oven perforated pan and top with the garlic cloves. Roast for about 25 minutes, or until the garlic is soft and the chicken reaches an internal temperature of 165ºF (74ºC) on a meat thermometer. Serve immediately.

Simple Chicken Shawarma

Prep time: 10 minutes | Cook time: 15 minutes | Serves 4

Shawarma Spice:

2 teaspoons dried oregano

1 teaspoon ground cinnamon

1 teaspoon ground cumin

1 teaspoon ground coriander

1 teaspoon kosher salt

½ teaspoon ground allspice

½ teaspoon cayenne pepper

Chicken:

1 pound (454 g) boneless, skinless chicken thighs, cut into large bite-size chunks

2 tablespoons vegetable oil

For Serving:

Tzatziki

Pita bread

1. For the shawarma spice: In a small bowl, combine the oregano, cayenne, cumin, coriander, salt, cinnamon, and allspice.

2. For the chicken: In a large bowl, toss together the chicken, vegetable oil, and shawarma spice to coat. Marinate at room temperature for 30 minutes or cover and refrigerate for up to 24 hours.

3. Set the temperature of the air fryer oven to 350ºF (177ºC). Press Start to begin preheating. Place the chicken in the air fryer oven perforated pan. Air fry for 15 minutes, or until the chicken reaches an internal temperature of 165ºF (74ºC).

4. Transfer the chicken to a serving platter. Serve with tzatziki and pita bread.

Spiced Turkey Tenderloin

Prep time: 20 minutes | Cook time: 30 minutes | Serves 4

½ teaspoon paprika

½ teaspoon garlic powder

½ teaspoon salt

½ teaspoon freshly ground black pepper

Pinch cayenne pepper

1½ pounds (680 g) turkey breast tenderloin

Olive oil spray

1. Set the temperature of the air fryer oven to 370ºF (188ºC). Press Start to begin preheating. Spray the air fryer oven perforated pan lightly with olive oil spray.

2. In a small bowl, combine the paprika, garlic powder, salt, black pepper, and cayenne pepper. Rub the mixture all over the turkey.

3. Place the turkey in the air fryer oven perforated pan and lightly spray with olive oil spray.

4. Air fry for 15 minutes. Flip the turkey over and lightly spray with olive oil spray. Air fry until the internal temperature reaches at least 170ºF (77ºC) for an additional 10 to 15 minutes.

5. Let the turkey rest for 10 minutes before slicing and serving.

Sweet and Spicy Turkey Meatballs

Prep time: 15 minutes | Cook time: 15 minutes | Serves 6

1 pound (454 g) lean ground turkey

½ cup whole-wheat panko bread crumbs

1 egg, beaten

1 tablespoon soy sauce

¼ cup plus 1 tablespoon hoisin sauce, divided

2 teaspoons minced garlic

⅛ teaspoon salt

⅛ teaspoon freshly ground black pepper

1 teaspoon sriracha

Cooking spray

1. Set the temperature of the air fryer oven to 350ºF (177ºC). Press Start to begin preheating. Spray the air fryer oven perforated pan lightly with cooking spray.

2. In a large bowl, mix together the turkey, panko bread crumbs, egg, soy sauce, 1 tablespoon of hoisin sauce, garlic, salt, and black pepper.

3. Using a tablespoon, form the mixture into 24 meatballs.

4. In a small bowl, combine the remaining ¼ cup of hoisin sauce and sriracha to make a glaze and set aside.

5. Place the meatballs in the air fryer oven perforated pan in a single layer. You may need to cook them in batches.

6. Air fry for 8 minutes. Brush the meatballs generously with the glaze and air fry until cooked through, an additional 4 to 7 minutes. Serve warm.

Sweet-and-Sour Drumsticks

Prep time: 5 minutes | Cook time: 23 to 25 minutes | Serves 4

6 chicken drumsticks

3 tablespoons lemon juice, divided

3 tablespoons low-sodium soy sauce, divided

1 tablespoon peanut oil

3 tablespoons honey

3 tablespoons brown sugar

2 tablespoons ketchup

¼ cup pineapple juice

1. Set the temperature of the air fryer oven to 350ºF (177ºC). Press Start to begin preheating.

2. Sprinkle the drumsticks with 1 tablespoon of lemon juice and 1 tablespoon of soy sauce. Place in the air fryer oven perforated pan and drizzle with the peanut oil. Toss to coat. Bake for 18 minutes or until the chicken is almost done.

3. Meanwhile, in a metal bowl combine the remaining 2 tablespoons of lemon juice, the remaining 2 tablespoons of soy sauce, honey, brown sugar, ketchup, and pineapple juice.

4. Add the cooked chicken to the bowl and stir to coat the chicken well with the sauce.

5. Place the metal bowl in the air fryer oven. Bake for 5 to 7 minutes or until the chicken is glazed and registers 165ºF (74ºC) on a meat thermometer.

6. Serve warm.

Tempero Baiano Brazilian Chicken

Prep time: 5 minutes | Cook time: 20 minutes | Serves 4

1 teaspoon cumin seeds

1 teaspoon dried oregano

1 teaspoon dried parsley

1 teaspoon ground turmeric

½ teaspoon coriander seeds

1 teaspoon kosher salt

½ teaspoon black peppercorns

½ teaspoon cayenne pepper

¼ cup fresh lime juice

2 tablespoons olive oil

1½ pounds (680 g) chicken drumsticks

1. In a clean coffee grinder or spice mill, combine the cumin, oregano, parsley, turmeric, coriander seeds, salt, peppercorns, and cayenne. Process until finely ground.

2. In a small bowl, combine the ground spices with the lime juice and oil. Place the chicken in a resealable plastic bag. Add the marinade, seal, and massage until the chicken is well coated. Marinate at room temperature for 30 minutes or in the refrigerator for up to 24 hours.

3. Set the temperature of the air fryer oven to 400ºF (204ºC). Press Start to begin preheating.

4. Place the drumsticks skin-side up in the air fryer oven perforated pan and air fry for 20 to 25 minutes, turning the drumsticks halfway through the cooking time. Use a meat thermometer to ensure that the chicken has reached an internal temperature of 165ºF (74ºC). Serve immediately.

Tex-Mex Chicken Breasts

Prep time: 10 minutes | Cook time: 17 to 20 minutes | Serves 4

1 pound (454 g) low-sodium boneless, skinless chicken breasts, cut into 1-inch cubes

1 medium onion, chopped

1 red bell pepper, chopped

1 jalapeño pepper, minced

2 teaspoons olive oil

$^2/_3$ cup canned low-sodium black beans, rinsed and drained

½ cup low-sodium salsa

2 teaspoons chili powder

1. Set the temperature of the air fryer oven to 400ºF (204ºC). Press Start to begin preheating.

2. In a medium metal bowl, mix the chicken, onion, bell pepper, jalapeño, and olive oil. Roast for 10 minutes, stirring once during cooking.

3. Add the black beans, salsa, and chili powder. Roast for 7 to 10 minutes more, stirring once, until the chicken reaches an internal temperature of 165ºF (74ºC) on a meat thermometer. Serve immediately.

Tex-Mex Turkey Burgers

Prep time: 10 minutes | Cook time: 14 to 16 minutes | Serves 4

$^1/_3$ cup finely crushed corn tortilla chips

1 egg, beaten

¼ cup salsa

$^1/_3$ cup shredded pepper Jack cheese

Pinch salt

Freshly ground black pepper, to taste

1 pound (454 g) ground turkey

1 tablespoon olive oil

1 teaspoon paprika

1. Set the temperature of the air fryer oven to 330ºF (166ºC). Press Start to begin preheating.

2. In a medium bowl, combine the tortilla chips, egg, salsa, cheese, salt, and pepper, and mix well.

3. Add the turkey and mix gently but thoroughly with clean hands.

4. Form the meat mixture into patties about ½ inch thick. Make an indentation in the center of each patty with the thumb so the burgers don't puff up while cooking.

5. Brush the patties on both sides with the olive oil and sprinkle with paprika.

6. Put in the air fryer oven perforated pan and air fry for 14 to 16 minutes or until the meat registers at least 165ºF (74ºC).

7. Let sit for 5 minutes before serving.

Thai Cornish Game Hens

Prep time: 15 minutes | Cook time: 20 minutes | Serves 4

1 cup chopped fresh cilantro leaves and stems

¼ cup fish sauce

1 tablespoon soy sauce

1 serrano chile, seeded and chopped

8 garlic cloves, smashed

2 tablespoons sugar

2 tablespoons lemongrass paste

2 teaspoons black pepper

2 teaspoons ground coriander

1 teaspoon kosher salt

1 teaspoon ground turmeric

2 Cornish game hens, giblets removed, split in half lengthwise

1. In a blender, combine the cilantro, fish sauce, soy sauce, serrano, garlic, sugar, lemongrass, black pepper, coriander, salt, and turmeric. Blend until smooth.

2. Place the game hen halves in a large bowl. Pour the cilantro mixture over the hen halves and toss to coat. Marinate at room temperature for 30 minutes, or cover and refrigerate for up to 24 hours.

3. Set the temperature of the air fryer oven to 400ºF (204ºC). Press Start to begin preheating.

4. Arrange the hen halves in a single layer in the air fryer oven perforated pan. Roast for 20 minutes. Use a meat thermometer to ensure the game hens have reached an internal temperature of 165ºF (74ºC). Serve warm.

Thai Curry Meatballs

Prep time: 10 minutes | Cook time: 10 minutes | Serves 4

1 pound (454 g) ground chicken

¼ cup chopped fresh cilantro

1 teaspoon chopped fresh mint

1 tablespoon fresh lime juice

1 tablespoon Thai red, green, or yellow curry paste

1 tablespoon fish sauce

2 garlic cloves, minced

2 teaspoons minced fresh ginger

½ teaspoon kosher salt

½ teaspoon black pepper

¼ teaspoon red pepper flakes

1. Set the temperature of the air fryer oven to 400ºF (204ºC). Press Start to begin preheating.

2. In a large bowl, gently mix the ground chicken, cilantro, mint, lime juice, curry paste, fish sauce, garlic, ginger, salt, black pepper, and red pepper flakes until thoroughly combined.

3. Form the mixture into 16 meatballs. Place the meatballs in a single layer in the air fryer oven perforated pan. Air fry for 10 minutes, turning the meatballs halfway through the cooking time. Use a meat thermometer to ensure the meatballs have reached an internal temperature of 165ºF (74ºC). Serve immediately.

Turkey and Cranberry Quesadillas

Prep time: 7 minutes | Cook time: 4 to 8 minutes | Serves 4

6 low-sodium whole-wheat tortillas

$^1/_3$ cup shredded low-sodium low-fat Swiss cheese

¾ cup shredded cooked low-sodium turkey breast

2 tablespoons cranberry sauce

2 tablespoons dried cranberries

½ teaspoon dried basil

Olive oil spray, for spraying the tortillas

1. Set the temperature of the air fryer oven to 400ºF (204ºC). Press Start to begin preheating.

2. Put 3 tortillas on a work surface.

3. Evenly divide the Swiss cheese, turkey, cranberry sauce, and dried cranberries among the tortillas. Sprinkle with the basil and top with the remaining tortillas.

4. Spray the outsides of the tortillas with olive oil spray.

5. One at a time, air fry the quesadillas in the air fryer oven for 4 to 8 minutes, or until crisp and the cheese is melted. Cut into quarters and serve.

Turkey Hoisin Burgers

Prep time: 10 minutes | Cook time: 20 minutes | Serves 4

1 pound (454 g) lean ground turkey

¼ cup whole-wheat bread crumbs

¼ cup hoisin sauce

2 tablespoons soy sauce

4 whole-wheat buns

Olive oil spray

1. In a large bowl, mix together the turkey, bread crumbs, hoisin sauce, and soy sauce.

2. Form the mixture into 4 equal patties. Cover with plastic wrap and refrigerate the patties for 30 minutes.

3. Set the temperature of the air fryer oven to 370ºF (188ºC). Press Start to begin preheating. Spray the air fryer oven perforated pan lightly with olive oil spray.

4. Place the patties in the air fryer oven perforated pan in a single layer. Spray the patties lightly with olive oil spray.

5. Air fry for 10 minutes. Flip the patties over, lightly spray with olive oil spray, and air fry for an additional 5 to 10 minutes, until golden brown.

6. Place the patties on buns and top with the choice of low-calorie burger toppings like sliced tomatoes, onions, and cabbage slaw. Serve immediately.

Turkey Stuffed Bell Peppers

Prep time: 20 minutes | Cook time: 15 minutes | Serves 4

½ pound (227 g) lean ground turkey

4 medium bell peppers

1 (15-ounce / 425-g) can black beans, drained and rinsed

1 cup shredded reduced-fat Cheddar cheese

1 cup cooked long-grain brown rice

1 cup mild salsa

1¼ teaspoons chili powder

1 teaspoon salt

½ teaspoon ground cumin

½ teaspoon freshly ground black pepper

Olive oil spray

Chopped fresh cilantro, for garnish

1. Set the temperature of the air fryer oven to 360ºF (182ºC). Press Start to begin preheating.

2. In a large skillet over medium-high heat, cook the turkey, breaking it up with a spoon, until browned, about 5 minutes. Drain off any excess fat.

3. Cut about ½ inch off the tops of the peppers and then cut in half lengthwise. Remove and discard the seeds and set the peppers aside.

89

4. In a large bowl, combine the browned turkey, black beans, Cheddar cheese, rice, salsa, chili powder, salt, cumin, and black pepper. Spoon the mixture into the bell peppers.

5. Lightly spray the air fryer oven perforated pan with olive oil spray.

6. Place the stuffed peppers in the air fryer oven perforated pan. Air fry until heated through, 10 to 15 minutes. Garnish with cilantro and serve.

Turkey, Hummus, and Cheese Wraps

Prep time: 10 minutes | Cook time: 3 to 4 minutes | Serves 4

4 large whole wheat wraps

½ cup hummus

16 thin slices deli turkey

8 slices provolone cheese

1 cup fresh baby spinach, or more to taste

1. Set the temperature of the air fryer oven to 360ºF (182ºC). Press Start to begin preheating.

2. To assemble, place 2 tablespoons of hummus on each wrap and spread to within about a half inch from edges. Top with 4 slices of turkey and 2 slices of provolone. Finish with ¼ cup of baby spinach, or pile on as much as you like.

3. Roll up each wrap. Place 2 wraps in air fryer oven perforated pan, seam-side down.

4. Air fry for 3 to 4 minutes to warm filling and melt cheese. Repeat step 4 to air fry the remaining wraps. Serve immediately.

Turkish Chicken Kebabs

Prep time: 15 minutes | Cook time: 15 minutes | Serves 4

¼ cup plain Greek yogurt

1 tablespoon minced garlic

1 tablespoon tomato paste

1 tablespoon fresh lemon juice

1 tablespoon vegetable oil

1 teaspoon kosher salt

1 teaspoon ground cumin

1 teaspoon sweet Hungarian paprika

½ teaspoon ground cinnamon

½ teaspoon black pepper

½ teaspoon cayenne pepper

1 pound (454 g) boneless, skinless chicken thighs, quartered crosswise

1. In a large bowl, combine the yogurt, garlic, tomato paste, lemon juice, vegetable oil, salt, cumin, paprika, cinnamon, black pepper, and cayenne. Stir until the spices are blended into the yogurt.

2. Add the chicken to the bowl and toss until well coated. Marinate at room temperature for 30 minutes, or cover and refrigerate for up to 24 hours.

3. Set the temperature of the air fryer oven to 375ºF (191ºC). Press Start to begin preheating.

4. Arrange the chicken in a single layer in the air fryer oven perforated pan. Air fry for 10 minutes. Turn the chicken and air fry for 5 minutes more. Use a meat thermometer to ensure the chicken has reached an internal temperature of 165ºF (74ºC).

5. Serve warm.

Yellow Curry Chicken Thighs with Peanuts

Prep time: 10 minutes | Cook time: 20 minutes | Serves 6

½ cup unsweetened full-fat coconut milk

2 tablespoons yellow curry paste

1 tablespoon minced fresh ginger

1 tablespoon minced garlic

1 teaspoon kosher salt

1 pound (454 g) boneless, skinless chicken thighs, halved crosswise

2 tablespoons chopped peanuts

1. In a large bowl, stir together the coconut milk, curry paste, ginger, garlic, and salt until well blended. Add the chicken; toss well to coat. Marinate at room temperature for 30 minutes, or cover and refrigerate for up to 24 hours.

2. Set the temperature of the air fryer oven to 375ºF (191ºC). Press Start to begin preheating.

3. Place the chicken (along with marinade) in a baking pan. Place the pan in the air fryer oven. Bake for 20 minutes, turning the chicken halfway through the cooking time. Use a meat thermometer to ensure the chicken has reached an internal temperature of 165ºF (74ºC).

4. Sprinkle the chicken with the chopped peanuts and serve.

Air Fried Spring Rolls

Prep time: 10 minutes | Cook time: 17 to 22 minutes | Serves 4

2 teaspoons minced garlic

2 cups finely sliced cabbage

1 cup matchstick cut carrots

2 (4-ounce / 113-g) cans tiny shrimp, drained

4 teaspoons soy sauce

Salt and freshly ground black pepper, to taste

16 square spring roll wrappers

Cooking spray

1. Set the temperature of the air fryer oven to 370ºF (188ºC). Press Start to begin preheating.

2. Spray the air fryer oven perforated pan lightly with cooking spray. Spray a medium sauté pan with cooking spray.

3. Add the garlic to the sauté pan and cook over medium heat until fragrant, 30 to 45 seconds. Add the cabbage and carrots and sauté until the vegetables are slightly tender, about 5 minutes.

4. Add the shrimp and soy sauce and season with salt and pepper, then stir to combine. Sauté until the moisture has evaporated, 2 more minutes. Set aside to cool.

5. Place a spring roll wrapper on a work surface so it looks like a diamond. Place 1 tablespoon of the shrimp mixture on the lower end of the wrapper.

6. Roll the wrapper away from you halfway, then fold in the right and left sides, like an envelope. Continue to roll to the very end, using a little water to seal the edge. Repeat with the remaining wrappers and filling.

7. Place the spring rolls in the air fryer perforated pan in a single layer, leaving room between each roll. Lightly spray with cooking spray. You may need to cook them in batches.

8. Air fry for 5 minutes. Turn the rolls over, lightly spray with cooking spray, and air fry until heated through and the rolls start to brown, 5 to 10 more minutes.

9. Cool for 5 minutes before serving.

Bacon-Wrapped Scallops

Prep time: 10 minutes | Cook time: 12 minutes | Serves 4

12 slices bacon

24 large sea scallops, tendons removed

1 teaspoon plus 2 tablespoons extra-virgin olive oil, divided

Salt and pepper, to taste

6 (6-inch) wooden skewers

1 tablespoon cider vinegar

1 teaspoon Dijon mustard

5 ounces (142 g) baby spinach

1 fennel bulb, stalks discarded, bulb halved, cored, and sliced thin

5 ounces (142 g) raspberries

1. Set the temperature of the air fryer oven to 350ºF (177ºC). Press Start to begin preheating.

2. Line large plate with 4 layers of paper towels and arrange 6 slices bacon over towels in a single layer. Top with 4 more layers of paper towels and remaining 6 slices bacon. Cover with 2 layers of paper towels, place a second large plate on top, and press gently to flatten. Microwave until fat begins to render but bacon is still pliable, about 5 minutes.

3. Pat scallops dry with paper towels and toss with 1 teaspoon oil, ⅛ teaspoon salt, and ⅛ teaspoon pepper in a bowl until evenly coated. Arrange 2 scallops side to

side, flat side down, on the cutting board. Starting at narrow end, wrap 1 slice bacon tightly around sides of scallop bundle. (Bacon should overlap slightly; trim excess as needed.) Thread scallop bundle onto skewer through bacon. Repeat with remaining scallops and bacon, threading 2 bundles onto each skewer.

4. Arrange 3 skewers in air fryer oven perforated pan, parallel to each other and spaced evenly apart. Arrange remaining 3 skewers on top, perpendicular to the bottom layer. Bake until bacon is crisp and scallops are firm and centers are opaque, 12 to 16 minutes, flipping and rotating skewers halfway through cooking.

5. Meanwhile, whisk remaining 2 tablespoons oil, vinegar, mustard, ⅛ teaspoon salt, and ⅛ teaspoon pepper in large serving bowl until combined. Add spinach, fennel, and raspberries and gently toss to coat. Serve skewers with salad.

Baja Fish Tacos

Prep time: 15 minutes | Cook time: 10 minutes | Serves 4

Fried Fish

1 pound (454 g) tilapia fillets (or other mild white fish)

½ cup all-purpose flour

1 teaspoon garlic powder

1 teaspoon kosher salt

¼ teaspoon cayenne pepper

½ cup mayonnaise

3 tablespoons milk

1¾ cups panko bread crumbs

Vegetable oil for spraying

Tacos

8 corn tortillas

¼ head red or green cabbage, shredded

1 ripe avocado, halved and each half cut into 4 slices

12 ounces (340 g) pico de gallo or other fresh salsa

Dollop of Mexican crema

1 lime, cut into wedges

1. To make the fish, cut the fish fillets into strips 3 to 4 inches long and 1 inch wide. Combine the flour, garlic powder, salt, and cayenne pepper on a plate and whisk to combine. In a shallow bowl, whisk the mayonnaise and milk together. Place the panko on a separate plate.

Dredge the fish strips in the seasoned flour, shaking off any excess. Dip the strips in the mayonnaise mixture, coating them completely, then dredge in the panko, shaking off any excess. Place the fish strips on a plate or rack.

2. Set the temperature of the air fryer oven to 400ºF (204ºC). Press Start to begin preheating. Working in batches, spray half the fish strips with oil and arrange them in the air fryer oven perforated pan, taking care not to crowd them. Air fry for 4 minutes, then flip and air fry for another 3 to 4 minutes until the outside is brown and crisp and the inside is opaque and flakes easily with a fork. Repeat with the remaining strips.

3. Heat the tortillas in the microwave or on the stovetop. To assemble the tacos, place 2 fish strips inside each tortilla. Top with shredded cabbage, a slice of avocado, pico de gallo, and a dollop of crema. Serve with a lime wedge on the side.

Better-Than-Boxed Fish Sticks

Prep time: 10 minutes | Cook time: 10 to 12 minutes | Serves 4

Salt and pepper, to taste

1½ pounds (680g) skinless haddock fillets, ¾ inch thick, sliced into 4-inch strips

2 cups panko bread crumbs

1 tablespoon vegetable oil

¼ cup all-purpose flour

¼ cup mayonnaise

2 large eggs

1 tablespoon Old Bay seasoning

Vegetable oil spray

1. Dissolve ¼ cup salt in 2 quarts cold water in large container. Add the haddock, cover, and let sit for 15 minutes.

2. Toss the panko with oil in a bowl until evenly coated. Microwave, stirring frequently, until light golden brown, 2 to 4 minutes; transfer to shallow dish. Whisk the flour, mayonnaise, eggs, mustard, Old Bay, ⅛ teaspoon salt, and ⅛ teaspoon pepper together in a second shallow dish.

3. Set a wire rack in a rimmed baking sheet and spray with vegetable oil spray. Remove the haddock from the brine and thoroughly pat dry with paper towels. Working with

1 piece at a time, dredge the haddock in the egg mixture, letting excess drip off, then coat with the panko mixture, pressing gently to adhere. Transfer the fish sticks to the prepared rack and freeze until firm, about 1 hour.

4. Set the temperature of the air fryer oven to 400ºF (204ºC). Press Start to begin preheating. Lightly spray the air fryer oven perforated pan with vegetable oil spray. Arrange up to 5 fish sticks in the prepared perforated pan, spaced evenly apart. Air fry until fish sticks are golden and register 140ºF (60ºC), 10 to 12 minutes, flipping and rotating fish sticks halfway through cooking.

5. Serve warm.

Blackened Fish

Prep time: 15 minutes | Cook time: 8 minutes | Serves 4

1 large egg, beaten

Blackened seasoning, as needed

2 tablespoons light brown sugar

4 (4-ounce / 113- g) tilapia fillets

Cooking spray

1. In a shallow bowl, place the beaten egg. In a second shallow bowl, stir together the Blackened seasoning and the brown sugar.

2. One at a time, dip the fish fillets in the egg, then the brown sugar mixture, coating thoroughly.

3. Set the temperature of the air fryer oven to 300ºF (149ºC). Press Start to begin preheating. Line the air fryer oven perforated pan with parchment paper.

4. Place the coated fish on the parchment and spritz with oil.

5. Bake for 4 minutes. Flip the fish, spritz it with oil, and bake for 4 to 6 minutes more until the fish is white inside and flakes easily with a fork.

6. Serve immediately.

Blackened Salmon

Prep time: 10 minutes | Cook time: 5 to 7 minutes | Serves 4

Salmon:

1 tablespoon sweet paprika

½ teaspoon cayenne pepper

1 teaspoon garlic powder

1 teaspoon dried oregano

1 teaspoon dried thyme

¾ teaspoon kosher salt

⅛ teaspoon freshly ground black pepper

Cooking spray

4 (6 ounces / 170 g each) wild salmon fillets

Cucumber-Avocado Salsa:

2 tablespoons chopped red onion

1½ tablespoons fresh lemon juice

1 teaspoon extra-virgin olive oil

¼ teaspoon plus ⅛ teaspoon kosher salt

Freshly ground black pepper, to taste

4 Persian cucumbers, diced

6 ounces (170 g) Hass avocado, diced

1. For the salmon: In a small bowl, combine the paprika, cayenne, garlic powder, oregano, thyme, salt, and black pepper. Spray both sides of the fish with oil and rub all over. Coat the fish all over with the spices.

2. For the cucumber-avocado salsa: In a medium bowl, combine the red onion, lemon juice, olive oil, salt, and pepper. Let stand for 5 minutes, then add the cucumbers and avocado.

3. Set the temperature of the air fryer oven to 400ºF (204ºC). Press Start to begin preheating.

4. Working in batches, arrange the salmon fillets skin side down in the air fryer oven perforated pan. Air fry for 5 to 7 minutes, or until the fish flakes easily with a fork, depending on the thickness of the fish.

5. Serve topped with the salsa.

Blackened Shrimp Tacos

Prep time: 10 minutes | Cook time: 10 to 15 minutes | Serves 4

1 teaspoon olive oil, plus more for spraying

12 ounces (340 g) medium shrimp, deveined, tails off

1 to 2 teaspoons blackened seasoning

8 corn tortillas, warmed

1 (14-ounce / 397-g) bag coleslaw mix

2 limes, cut in half

1. Set the temperature of the air fryer oven to 400ºF (204ºC). Press Start to begin preheating.

2. Spray the air fryer oven perforated pan lightly with cooking spray.

3. Dry the shrimp with a paper towel to remove excess water.

4. In a medium bowl, toss the shrimp with olive oil and Blackened seasoning.

5. Place the shrimp in the air fryer perforated pan and air fry for 5 minutes. Shake the perforated pan, lightly spray with cooking spray, and air fry until the shrimp are cooked through and starting to brown, 5 to 10 more minutes.

6. Fill each tortilla with the coleslaw mix and top with the blackened shrimp. Squeeze fresh lime juice over top and serve.

Cajun Fish Fillets

Prep time: 15 minutes | Cook time: 6 minutes | Serves 4

¾ cup all-purpose flour

¼ cup yellow cornmeal

1 large egg, beaten

¼ cup Cajun seasoning

4 (4-ounce / 113-g) catfish fillets

Cooking spray

1. In a shallow bowl, whisk the flour and cornmeal until blended. Place the egg in a second shallow bowl and the Cajun seasoning in a third shallow bowl.

2. One at a time, dip the catfish fillets in the breading, the egg, and the Cajun seasoning, coating thoroughly.

3. Set the temperature of the air fryer oven to 300ºF (149ºC). Press Start to begin preheating. Line the air fryer oven perforated pan with parchment paper.

4. Place the coated fish on the parchment and spritz with oil.

5. Bake for 3 minutes. Flip the fish, spritz it with oil, and bake for 3 to 5 minutes more until the fish flakes easily with a fork and reaches an internal temperature of 145ºF (63ºC). Serve warm.

Cajun-Style Fish Tacos

Prep time: 5 minutes | Cook time: 10 to 15 minutes | Serves 6

2 teaspoons avocado oil

1 tablespoon Cajun seasoning

4 tilapia fillets

1 (14-ounce / 397-g) package coleslaw mix

12 corn tortillas

2 limes, cut into wedges

1. Set the temperature of the air fryer oven to 380ºF (193ºC). Press Start to begin preheating. Line the air fryer oven perforated pan with parchment paper.

2. In a medium, shallow bowl mix the avocado oil and the Cajun seasoning to make a marinade. Add the tilapia fillets and coat evenly.

3. Place the fillets in the perforated pan in a single layer, leaving room between each fillet. You may need to cook in batches.

4. Air fry until the fish is cooked and easily flakes with a fork, 10 to 15 minutes.

5. Assemble the tacos by placing some of the coleslaw mix in each tortilla. Add $^1/_3$ of a tilapia fillet to each tortilla. Squeeze some lime juice over the top of each taco and serve.

Cajun-Style Salmon Burgers

Prep time: 10 minutes | Cook time: 10 to 15 minutes | Serves 4

4 (5-ounce / 142-g) cans pink salmon in water, any skin and bones removed, drained

2 eggs, beaten

1 cup whole-wheat bread crumbs

4 tablespoons light mayonnaise

2 teaspoons Cajun seasoning

2 teaspoons dry mustard

4 whole-wheat buns

Cooking spray

1. In a medium bowl, mix the salmon, egg, bread crumbs, mayonnaise, Cajun seasoning, and dry mustard. Cover with plastic wrap and refrigerate for 30 minutes.

2. Set the temperature of the air fryer oven to 360ºF (182ºC). Press Start to begin preheating. Spray the air fryer oven perforated pan lightly with cooking spray.

3. Shape the mixture into four ½-inch-thick patties about the same size as the buns.

4. Place the salmon patties in the perforated pan in a single layer and lightly spray the tops with cooking spray. You may need to cook them in batches.

5. Air fry for 6 to 8 minutes. Turn the patties over and lightly spray with cooking spray. Air fry until crispy on the outside, 4 to 7 more minutes.

6. Serve on whole-wheat buns.

Apple, Peach, and Cranberry Crisp

Prep time: 10 minutes | Cook time: 12 minutes | Serves 8

1 apple, peeled and chopped

2 peaches, peeled and chopped

⅓ cup dried cranberries

2 tablespoons honey

⅓ cup brown sugar

¼ cup flour

½ cup oatmeal

3 tablespoons softened butter

1. Set the temperature of the air fryer oven to 370ºF (188ºC). Press Start to begin preheating.

2. In a baking pan, combine the apple, peaches, cranberries, and honey, and mix well.

3. In a medium bowl, combine the brown sugar, flour, oatmeal, and butter, and mix until crumbly. Sprinkle this mixture over the fruit in the pan.

4. Bake for 10 to 12 minutes or until the fruit is bubbly and the topping is golden brown. Serve warm.

Applesauce and Chocolate Brownies

Prep time: 10 minutes | Cook time: 15 minutes | Serves 8

¼ cup unsweetened cocoa powder

¼ cup all-purpose flour

¼ teaspoon kosher salt

½ teaspoons baking powder

3 tablespoons unsalted butter, melted

½ cup granulated sugar

1 large egg

3 tablespoons unsweetened applesauce

¼ cup miniature semisweet chocolate chips

Coarse sea salt, to taste

1. Set the temperature of the air fryer oven to 300ºF (149ºC). Press Start to begin preheating.

2. In a large bowl, whisk together the cocoa powder, all-purpose flour, kosher salt, and baking powder.

3. In a separate large bowl, combine the butter, granulated sugar, egg, and applesauce, then use a spatula to fold in the cocoa powder mixture and the chocolate chips until well combined.

4. Spray a baking pan with nonstick cooking spray, then pour the mixture into the pan. Place the pan in the air

fryer oven and bake for 15 minutes or until a toothpick comes out clean when inserted in the middle.

5. Remove the brownies from the air fryer oven, sprinkle some coarse sea salt on top, and allow to cool in the pan on a wire rack for 20 minutes before cutting and serving.

Baked Apples

Prep time: 5 minutes | Cook time: 10 minutes | Serves 4

4 small apples, cored and cut in half

2 tablespoons salted butter or coconut oil, melted

2 tablespoons sugar

1 teaspoon apple pie spice

Ice cream, heavy cream, or whipped cream, for serving

1. Set the temperature of the air fryer oven to 350ºF (177ºC). Press Start to begin preheating.

2. Put the apples in a large bowl. Drizzle with the melted butter and sprinkle with the sugar and apple pie spice. Use the hands to toss, ensuring the apples are evenly coated.

3. Put the apples in the air fryer oven perforated pan and bake for 10 minutes. Pierce the apples with a fork to ensure they are tender.

4. Serve with ice cream, or top with a splash of heavy cream or a spoonful of whipped cream.

Banana and Walnut Cake

Prep time: 10 minutes | Cook time: 10 minutes | Serves 6

1 pound (454 g) bananas, mashed

8 ounces (227 g) flour

6 ounces (170 g) sugar

3.5 ounces (99 g) walnuts, chopped

2.5 ounces (71 g) butter

2 eggs

¼ teaspoon baking soda

1. Coat the inside of a baking dish with a little oil.

2. Set the temperature of the air fryer oven to 355ºF (179ºC). Press Start to begin preheating.

3. In a bowl combine the sugar, butter, egg, flour and soda using a whisk. Throw in the bananas and walnuts.

4. Transfer the mixture to the dish. Put the dish in the air fryer oven and bake for 10 minutes.

5. Reduce the temperature to 330ºF (166ºC) and bake for another 15 minutes. Serve hot.

Berry Crumble

Prep time: 10 minutes | Cook time: 15 minutes | Serves 4

For the Filling:

2 cups mixed berries

2 tablespoons sugar

1 tablespoon cornstarch

1 tablespoon fresh lemon juice

For the Toppin g :

¼ cup all-purpose flour

¼ cup rolled oats

1 tablespoon sugar

2 tablespoons cold unsalted butter, cut into small cubes

Whipped cream or ice cream (optional)

1. Set the temperature of the air fryer oven to 400ºF (204ºC). Press Start to begin preheating.

2. For the filling: In a round baking pan, gently mix the berries, sugar, cornstarch, and lemon juice until thoroughly combined.

3. For the topping: In a small bowl, combine the flour, oats, and sugar. Stir the butter into the flour mixture until the mixture has the consistency of bread crumbs.

4. Sprinkle the topping over the berries.

5. Put the pan in the air fryer oven and air fry for 15 minutes. Let cool for 5 minutes on a wire rack.

6. Serve topped with whipped cream or ice cream, if desired.

Black Forest Pies

Prep time: 10 minutes | Cook time: 15 minutes | Serves 6

3 tablespoons milk or dark chocolate chips

2 tablespoons thick, hot fudge sauce

2 tablespoons chopped dried cherries

1 (10-by-15-inch) sheet puff pastry, thawed

1 egg white, beaten

2 tablespoons sugar

½ teaspoon cinnamon

1. Set the temperature of the air fryer oven to 350ºF (177ºC). Press Start to begin preheating.

2. In a small bowl, combine the chocolate chips, fudge sauce, and dried cherries.

3. Roll out the puff pastry on a floured surface. Cut into 6 squares with a sharp knife.

4. Divide the chocolate chip mixture into the center of each puff pastry square. Fold the squares in half to make triangles. Firmly press the edges with the tines of a fork to seal.

5. Brush the triangles on all sides sparingly with the beaten egg white. Sprinkle the tops with sugar and cinnamon.

6. Put in the air fryer oven perforated pan and bake for 15 minutes or until the triangles are golden brown. The filling will be hot, so cool for at least 20 minutes before serving.

Bourbon Bread Pudding

Prep time: 10 minutes | Cook time: 20 minutes | Serves 4

3 slices whole grain bread, cubed

1 large egg

1 cup whole milk

2 tablespoons bourbon

½ teaspoons vanilla extract

¼ cup maple syrup, divided

½ teaspoons ground cinnamon

2 teaspoons sparkling sugar

1. Set the temperature of the air fryer oven to 270ºF (132ºC). Press Start to begin preheating.

2. Spray a baking pan with nonstick cooking spray, then place the bread cubes in the pan.

3. In a medium bowl, whisk together the egg, milk, bourbon, vanilla extract, 3 tablespoons of maple syrup, and cinnamon. Pour the egg mixture over the bread and press down with a spatula to coat all the bread, then sprinkle the sparkling sugar on top and bake for 20 minutes.

4. Remove the pudding from the air fryer oven and allow to cool in the pan on a wire rack for 10 minutes. Drizzle the remaining 1 tablespoon of maple syrup on top. Slice and serve warm.

Brazilian Pineapple Bake

Prep time: 5 minutes | Cook time: 16 minutes | Serves 4

½ cup brown sugar

2 teaspoons ground cinnamon

1 small pineapple, peeled, cored, and cut into spears

3 tablespoons unsalted butter, melted

1. Set the temperature of the air fryer oven to 400ºF (204ºC). Press Start to begin preheating.

2. In a small bowl, mix the brown sugar and cinnamon until thoroughly combined.

3. Brush the pineapple spears with the melted butter. Sprinkle the cinnamon-sugar over the spears, pressing lightly to ensure it adheres well.

4. Put the spears in the air fryer oven perforated pan in a single layer. (Depending on the size of the air fryer oven, you may have to do this in batches.) Bake for 10 minutes for the first batch (6 to 8 minutes for the next batch, as the air fryer oven will be preheated). Halfway through the cooking time, brush the spears with butter.

5. The pineapple spears are done when they are heated through and the sugar is bubbling. Serve hot.

Cardamom and Vanilla Custard

Prep time: 5 minutes | Cook time: 25 minutes | Serves 2

1 cup whole milk

1 large egg

2 tablespoons plus 1 teaspoon sugar

¼ teaspoon vanilla bean paste or pure vanilla extract

¼ teaspoon ground cardamom, plus more for sprinkling

1. Set the temperature of the air fryer oven to 350ºF (177ºC). Press Start to begin preheating.

2. In a medium bowl, beat together the milk, egg, sugar, vanilla, and cardamom.

3. Put two ramekins in the air fryer oven perforated pan. Divide the mixture between the ramekins. Sprinkle lightly with cardamom. Cover each ramekin tightly with aluminum foil. Bake for 25 minutes, or until a toothpick inserted in the center comes out clean.

4. Let the custards cool on a wire rack for 5 to 10 minutes.

5. Serve warm, or refrigerate until cold and serve chilled.

Chickpea Brownies

Prep time: 10 minutes | Cook time: 20 minutes | Serves 6

Vegetable oil

1 (15-ounce / 425-g) can chickpeas, drained and rinsed

4 large eggs

⅓ cup coconut oil, melted

⅓ cup honey

3 tablespoons unsweetened cocoa powder

1 tablespoon espresso powder (optional)

1 teaspoon baking powder

1 teaspoon baking soda

½ cup chocolate chips

1. Set the temperature of the air fryer oven to 325ºF (163ºC). Press Start to begin preheating.

2. Generously grease a baking pan with vegetable oil.

3. In a blender or food processor, combine the chickpeas, eggs, coconut oil, honey, cocoa powder, espresso powder (if using), baking powder, and baking soda. Blend or process until smooth. Transfer to the prepared pan and stir in the chocolate chips by hand.

4. Set the pan in the air fryer oven and bake for 20 minutes, or until a toothpick inserted into the center comes out clean.

5. Let cool in the pan on a wire rack for 30 minutes before cutting into squares.

6. Serve immediately.

Chocolate and Peanut Butter Lava Cupcakes

Prep time: 10 minutes | Cook time: 10 to 13 minutes | Serves 8

Nonstick baking spray with flour

$1^1/_3$ cups chocolate cake mix

1 egg

1 egg yolk

¼ cup safflower oil

¼ cup hot water

$^1/_3$ cup sour cream

3 tablespoons peanut butter

1 tablespoon powdered sugar

1. Set the temperature of the air fryer oven to 350ºF (177ºC). Press Start to begin preheating.

2. Double up 16 foil muffin cups to make 8 cups. Spray each lightly with nonstick spray; set aside.

3. In a medium bowl, combine the cake mix, egg, egg yolk, safflower oil, water, and sour cream, and beat until combined.

4. In a small bowl, combine the peanut butter and powdered sugar and mix well. Form this mixture into 8 balls.

5. Spoon about ¼ cup of the chocolate batter into each muffin cup and top with a peanut butter ball. Spoon remaining batter on top of the peanut butter balls to cover them.

6. Arrange the cups in the air fryer oven perforated pan, leaving some space between each. Bake for 10 to 13 minutes or until the tops look dry and set.

7. Let the cupcakes cool for about 10 minutes, then serve warm.

Chocolate Cake

Prep time: 10 minutes | Cook time: 55 minutes | Serves 4

Unsalted butter, at room temperature

3 large eggs

1 cup almond flour

⅔ cup sugar

⅓ cup heavy cream

¼ cup coconut oil, melted

¼ cup unsweetened cocoa powder

1 teaspoon baking powder

¼ cup chopped walnuts

1. Set the temperature of the air fryer oven to 400ºF (204ºC). Press Start to begin preheating.

2. Generously butter a round baking pan. Line the bottom of the pan with parchment paper cut to fit.

3. In a large bowl, combine the eggs, almond flour, sugar, cream, coconut oil, cocoa powder, and baking powder. Beat with a hand mixer on medium speed until well blended and fluffy. (This will keep the cake from being too dense, as almond flour cakes can sometimes be.) Fold in the walnuts.

4. Pour the batter into the prepared pan. Cover the pan tightly with aluminum foil. Set the pan in the air fryer oven and bake for 45 minutes. Remove the foil and bake for 10 to 15 minutes more until a knife (do not use a toothpick) inserted into the center of the cake comes out clean.

5. Let the cake cool in the pan on a wire rack for 10 minutes. Remove the cake from the pan and let cool on the rack for 20 minutes before slicing and serving.

Chocolate Coconut Brownies

Prep time: 15 minutes | Cook time: 15 minutes | Serves 8

½ cup coconut oil

2 ounces (57 g) dark chocolate

1 cup sugar

2½ tablespoons water

4 whisked eggs

¼ teaspoon ground cinnamon

½ teaspoons ground anise star

¼ teaspoon coconut extract

½ teaspoons vanilla extract

1 tablespoon honey

½ cup flour

½ cup desiccated coconut

Sugar, for dusting

1. Set the temperature of the air fryer oven to 355ºF (179ºC). Press Start to begin preheating.

2. Melt the coconut oil and dark chocolate in the microwave.

3. Combine with the sugar, water, eggs, cinnamon, anise, coconut extract, vanilla, and honey in a large bowl.

4. Stir in the flour and desiccated coconut. Incorporate everything well.

5. Lightly grease a baking dish with butter. Transfer the mixture to the dish.

6. Put the dish in the air fryer oven and bake for 15 minutes.

7. Remove from the air fryer oven and allow to cool slightly.

8. Take care when taking it out of the baking dish. Slice it into squares.

9. Dust with sugar before serving.

Chocolate Croissants

Prep time: 5 minutes | Cook time: 24 minutes | Serves 8

1 sheet frozen puff pastry, thawed

⅓ cup chocolate-hazelnut spread

1 large egg, beaten

1. On a lightly floured surface, roll puff pastry into a 14-inch square. Cut pastry into quarters to form 4 squares. Cut each square diagonally to form 8 triangles.

2. Spread 2 teaspoons chocolate-hazelnut spread on each triangle; from wider end, roll up pastry. Brush egg on top of each roll.

3. Set the temperature of the air fryer oven to 375ºF (191ºC). Press Start to begin preheating. Air fry rolls in batches, 3 or 4 at a time, 8 minutes per batch, or until pastry is golden brown.

4. Cool on a wire rack; serve while warm or at room temperature.

Chocolate Molten Cake

Prep time: 5 minutes | Cook time: 10 minutes | Serves 4

3.5 ounces (99 g) butter, melted

3½ tablespoons sugar

3.5 ounces (99 g) chocolate, melted

1½ tablespoons flour

2 eggs

1. Set the temperature of the air fryer oven to 375ºF (191ºC). Press Start to begin preheating.

2. Grease four ramekins with a little butter.

3. Rigorously combine the eggs, butter, and sugar before stirring in the melted chocolate.

4. Slowly fold in the flour.

5. Spoon an equal amount of the mixture into each ramekin.

6. Put them in the air fryer oven and bake for 10 minutes

7. Put the ramekins upside-down on plates and let the cakes fall out. Serve hot.

Chocolate S'mores

Prep time: 5 minutes | Cook time: 3 minutes | Serves 12

12 whole cinnamon graham crackers

2 (1.55-ounce / 44-g) chocolate bars, broken into 12 pieces

12 marshmallows

1. Set the temperature of the air fryer oven to 350ºF (177ºC). Press Start to begin preheating.

2. Halve each graham cracker into 2 squares.

3. Put 6 graham cracker squares in the air fryer oven. Do not stack. Put a piece of chocolate into each. Bake for 2 minutes.

4. Open the air fryer oven and add a marshmallow onto each piece of melted chocolate. Bake for 1 additional minute.

5. Remove the cooked s'mores from the air fryer oven, then repeat steps 2 and 3 for the remaining 6 s'mores.

6. Top with the remaining graham cracker squares and serve.

Cinnamon Almonds

Prep time: 5 minutes | Cook time: 8 minutes | Serves 4

1 cup whole almonds

2 tablespoons salted butter, melted

1 tablespoon sugar

½ teaspoon ground cinnamon

1. Set the temperature of the air fryer oven to 300ºF (149ºC). Press Start to begin preheating.

2. In a medium bowl, combine the almonds, butter, sugar, and cinnamon. Mix well to ensure all the almonds are coated with the spiced butter.

3. Transfer the almonds to the air fryer oven perforated pan and shake so they are in a single layer. Bake for 8 minutes, stirring the almonds halfway through the cooking time.

4. Let cool completely before serving.

Cinnamon and Pecan Pie

Prep time: 10 minutes | Cook time: 25 minutes | Serves 4

1 pie dough

½ teaspoons cinnamon

¾ teaspoon vanilla extract

2 eggs

¾ cup maple syrup

⅛ teaspoon nutmeg

3 tablespoons melted butter, divided

2 tablespoons sugar

½ cup chopped pecans

1. Set the temperature of the air fryer oven to 370ºF (188ºC). Press Start to begin preheating.

2. In a small bowl, coat the pecans in 1 tablespoon of melted butter.

3. Transfer the pecans to the air fryer oven and allow them to toast for about 10 minutes.

4. Put the pie dough in a greased pie pan and add the pecans on top.

5. In a bowl, mix the rest of the ingredients. Pour this over the pecans.

6. Put the pan in the air fryer oven and bake for 25 minutes.

7. Serve immediately.

Curry Peaches, Pears, and Plums

Prep time: 5 minutes | Cook time: 5 minutes | Serves 6 to 8

2 peaches

2 firm pears

2 plums

2 tablespoons melted butter

1 tablespoon honey

2 to 3 teaspoons curry powder

1. Set the temperature of the air fryer oven to 325ºF (163ºC). Press Start to begin preheating.

2. Cut the peaches in half, remove the pits, and cut each half in half again. Cut the pears in half, core them, and remove the stem. Cut each half in half again. Do the same with the plums.

3. Spread a large sheet of heavy-duty foil on the work surface. Arrange the fruit on the foil and drizzle with the butter and honey. Sprinkle with the curry powder.

4. Wrap the fruit in the foil, making sure to leave some air space in the packet.

5. Put the foil package in the perforated pan and bake for 5 to 8 minutes, shaking the perforated pan once during the cooking time, until the fruit is soft.

1. Serve immediately.

Easy Almond Shortbread

Prep time: 5 minutes | Cook time: 12 minutes | Serves 8

½ cup (1 stick) unsalted butter

½ cup sugar

1 teaspoon pure almond extract

1 cup all-purpose flour

1. Set the temperature of the air fryer oven to 375ºF (191ºC). Press Start to begin preheating.

2. In a bowl of a stand mixer fitted with the paddle attachment, beat the butter and sugar on medium speed until fluffy, 3 to 4 minutes. Add the almond extract and beat until combined, about 30 seconds. Turn the mixer to low. Add the flour a little at a time and beat for about 2 minutes more until well incorporated.

3. Pat the dough into an even layer in a round baking pan. Put the pan in the air fryer oven and bake for 12 minutes.

4. Carefully remove the pan from air fryer oven. While the shortbread is still warm and soft, cut it into 8 wedges.

5. Let cool in the pan on a wire rack for 5 minutes. Remove the wedges from the pan and let cool on the rack before serving.

Easy Chocolate Donuts

Prep time: 5 minutes | Cook time: 8 minutes | Serves 8

1 (8-ounce / 227-g) can jumbo biscuits

Cooking oil

Chocolate sauce, for drizzling

1. Set the temperature of the air fryer oven to 375ºF (191ºC)

2. Separate the biscuit dough into 8 biscuits and place them on a flat work surface. Use a small circle cookie cutter or a biscuit cutter to cut a hole in the center of each biscuit. You can also cut the holes using a knife.

3. Spray the air fryer oven perforated pan with cooking oil.

4. Put 4 donuts in the air fryer oven. Do not stack. Spray with cooking oil. Air fry for 4 minutes.

5. Open the air fryer oven and flip the donuts. Air fry for an additional 4 minutes.

6. Remove the cooked donuts from the air fryer oven, then repeat steps 3 and 4 for the remaining 4 donuts.

7. Drizzle chocolate sauce over the donuts and enjoy while warm.

Lemony Apple Butter

Prep time: 10 minutes | Cook time: 1 hour | Makes 1¼ cups

Cooking spray

2 cups unsweetened applesauce

⅔ cup packed light brown sugar

3 tablespoons fresh lemon juice

½ teaspoon kosher salt

¼ teaspoon ground cinnamon

⅛ teaspoon ground allspice

1. Set the temperature of the air fryer oven to 340ºF (171ºC). Press Start to begin preheating.

2. Spray a metal cake pan with cooking spray. Whisk together all the ingredients in a bowl until smooth, then pour into the greased pan. Set the pan in the air fryer oven and bake until the apple mixture is caramelized, reduced to a thick purée, and fragrant, about 1 hour.

3. Remove the pan from the air fryer oven, stir to combine the caramelized bits at the edge with the rest, then let cool completely to thicken.

4. Serve immediately.

Fried Golden Bananas

Prep time: 5 minutes | Cook time: 7 minutes | Serves 6

1 large egg

¼ cup cornstarch

¼ cup plain bread crumbs

3 bananas, halved crosswise

Cooking oil

Chocolate sauce, for drizzling

1. Set the temperature of the air fryer oven to 350ºF (177ºC). Press Start to begin preheating.

2. In a small bowl, beat the egg. In another bowl, place the cornstarch. Put the bread crumbs in a third bowl.

3. Dip the bananas in the cornstarch, then the egg, and then the bread crumbs.

4. Spray the air fryer oven perforated pan with cooking oil.

5. Put the bananas in the perforated pan and spray them with cooking oil. Air fry for 5 minutes.

6. Open the air fryer oven and flip the bananas. Air fry for an additional 2 minutes.

7. Transfer the bananas to plates. Drizzle the chocolate sauce over the bananas, and serve.

Graham Cracker Cheesecake

Prep time: 10 minutes | Cook time: 20 minutes | Serves 8

1 cup graham cracker crumbs

3 tablespoons softened butter

1½ (8-ounce / 227-g) packages cream cheese, softened

$^1/_3$ cup sugar

2 eggs, beaten

1 tablespoon flour

1 teaspoon vanilla

¼ cup chocolate syrup

1. Set the temperature of the air fryer oven to 450ºF (232ºC). Press Start to begin preheating.

2. For the crust, combine the graham cracker crumbs and butter in a small bowl and mix well. Press into the bottom of a baking pan and put in the freezer to set.

3. For the filling, combine the cream cheese and sugar in a medium bowl and mix well. Beat in the eggs, one at a time. Add the flour and vanilla.

4. Remove $^2/_3$ cup of the filling to a small bowl and stir in the chocolate syrup until combined.

5. Pour the vanilla filling into the pan with the crust. Drop the chocolate filling over the vanilla filling by the spoonful. With a clean butter knife, stir the fillings in a zigzag pattern to marbleize them.

6. Bake for 20 minutes or until the cheesecake is just set.

7. Cool on a wire rack for 1 hour, then chill in the refrigerator until the cheesecake is firm.

8. Serve immediately.

Honey-Roasted Pears

Prep time: 5 minutes | Cook time: 20 minutes | Serves 4

2 large Bosc pears, halved and deseeded

3 tablespoons honey

1 tablespoon unsalted butter

½ teaspoon ground cinnamon

¼ cup walnuts, chopped

¼ cup part skim low-fat ricotta cheese, divided

1. Set the temperature of the air fryer oven to 350ºF (180ºC). Press Start to begin preheating.

2. In a baking pan, place the pears, cut-side up.

3. In a small microwave-safe bowl, melt the honey, butter, and cinnamon. Brush this mixture over the cut sides of the pears.

4. Pour 3 tablespoons of water around the pears in the pan. Roast the pears in the preheated air fryer oven for 20 minutes, or until tender when pierced with a fork and slightly crisp on the edges, basting once with the liquid in the pan.

5. Carefully remove the pears from the pan and place on a serving plate. Drizzle each with some liquid from the pan, sprinkle the walnuts on top, and serve with a spoonful of ricotta cheese.

6. Serve immediately.

Jelly Doughnuts

Prep time: 5 minutes | Cook time: 5 minutes | Serves 8

1 (16.3-ounce / 462-g) package large refrigerator biscuits

Cooking spray

1¼ cups good-quality raspberry jam

Confectioners' sugar, for dusting

1. Set the temperature of the air fryer oven to 350ºF (177ºC). Press Start to begin preheating.

2. Separate biscuits into 8 rounds. Spray both sides of rounds lightly with oil.

3. Spray the perforated pan with oil and place 3 to 4 rounds in the perforated pan. Air fry for 5 minutes, or until golden brown. Transfer to a wire rack; let cool. Repeat with the remaining rounds.

4. Fill a pastry bag, fitted with small plain tip, with raspberry jam; use tip to poke a small hole in the side of each doughnut, then fill the centers with the jam. Dust doughnuts with confectioners' sugar.

5. Serve immediately.

Lemony Blackberry Crisp

Prep time: 5 minutes | Cook time: 20 minutes | Serves 1

2 tablespoons lemon juice

$^1/_3$ cup powdered erythritol

¼ teaspoon xantham gum

2 cup blackberries

1 cup crunchy granola

1. Set the temperature of the air fryer oven to 350ºF (177ºC). Press Start to begin preheating.

2. In a bowl, combine the lemon juice, erythritol, xantham gum, and blackberries. Transfer to a round baking dish and cover with aluminum foil.

3. Put the dish in the air fryer oven and bake for 12 minutes.

4. Take care when removing the dish from the air fryer oven. Give the blackberries a stir and top with the granola.

5. Return the dish to the air fryer oven and bake for an additional 3 minutes, this time at 320ºF (160ºC). Serve once the granola has turned brown and enjoy.

Oatmeal and Carrot Cookie Cups

Prep time: 10 minutes | Cook time: 8 minutes | Makes 16 cups

3 tablespoons unsalted butter, at room temperature

¼ cup packed brown sugar

1 tablespoon honey

1 egg white

½ teaspoon vanilla extract

⅓ cup finely grated carrot

½ cup quick-cooking oatmeal

⅓ cup whole-wheat pastry flour

½ teaspoon baking soda

¼ cup dried cherries

1. Set the temperature of the air fryer oven to 350ºF (177ºC)

2. In a medium bowl, beat the butter, brown sugar, and honey until well combined.

3. Add the egg white, vanilla, and carrot. Beat to combine.

4. Stir in the oatmeal, pastry flour, and baking soda.

5. Stir in the dried cherries.

6. Double up 32 mini muffin foil cups to make 16 cups. Fill each with about 4 teaspoons of dough. Bake the cookie cups, 8 at a time, for 8 minutes, or until light golden brown and just set. Serve warm.

Oatmeal Raisin Bars

Prep time: 15 minutes | Cook time: 15 minutes | Serves 8

$^1/_3$ cup all-purpose flour

¼ teaspoon kosher salt

¼ teaspoon baking powder

¼ teaspoon ground cinnamon

¼ cup light brown sugar, lightly packed

¼ cup granulated sugar

½ cup canola oil

1 large egg

1 teaspoon vanilla extract

1⅓ cups quick-cooking oats

$1/_3$ cup raisins

1. Set the temperature of the air fryer oven to 360ºF (182ºC). Press Start to begin preheating.

2. In a large bowl, combine the all-purpose flour, kosher salt, baking powder, ground cinnamon, light brown sugar, granulated sugar, canola oil, egg, vanilla extract, quick-cooking oats, and raisins.

3. Spray a baking pan with nonstick cooking spray, then pour the oat mixture into the pan and press down to evenly distribute. Place the pan in the air fryer oven and bake for 15 minutes or until golden brown.

4. Remove from the air fryer oven and allow to cool in the pan on a wire rack for 20 minutes before slicing and serving.

Orange Cake

Prep time: 10 minutes | Cook time: 23 minutes | Serves 8

Nonstick baking spray with flour

1¼ cups all-purpose flour

$^1/_3$ cup yellow cornmeal

¾ cup white sugar

1 teaspoon baking soda

¼ cup safflower oil

1¼ cups orange juice, divided

1 teaspoon vanilla

¼ cup powdered sugar

1. Set the temperature of the air fryer oven to 350ºF (177ºC). Press Start to begin preheating.

2. Spray a baking pan with nonstick spray and set aside.

3. In a medium bowl, combine the flour, cornmeal, sugar, baking soda, safflower oil, 1 cup of the orange juice, and vanilla, and mix well.

4. Pour the batter into the baking pan and place in the air fryer oven. Bake for 23 minutes or until a toothpick inserted in the center of the cake comes out clean.

5. Remove the cake from the oven and place on a cooling rack. Using a toothpick, make about 20 holes in the cake.

6. In a small bowl, combine remaining ¼ cup of orange juice and the powdered sugar and stir well. Drizzle this mixture over the hot cake slowly so the cake absorbs it.

7. Cool completely, then cut into wedges to serve.

Pear and Apple Crisp

Prep time: 10 minutes | Cook time: 20 minutes | Serves 6

½ pound (227 g) apples, cored and chopped

½ pound (227 g) pears, cored and chopped

1 cup flour

1 cup sugar

1 tablespoon butter

1 teaspoon ground cinnamon

¼ teaspoon ground cloves

1 teaspoon vanilla extract

¼ cup chopped walnuts

Whipped cream, for serving

1. Set the temperature of the air fryer oven to 340ºF (171ºC). Press Start to begin preheating.

2. Lightly grease a baking dish and place the apples and pears inside.

3. Combine the rest of the ingredients, minus the walnuts and the whipped cream, until a coarse, crumbly texture is achieved.

4. Pour the mixture over the fruits and spread it evenly. Top with the chopped walnuts.

5. Bake for 20 minutes or until the top turns golden brown.

6. When cooked through, serve at room temperature with whipped cream.

Pecan and Cherry Stuffed Apples

Prep time: 10 minutes | Cook time: 20 minutes | Serves 4

4 apples (about 1¼ pounds / 567 g)

¼ cup chopped pecans

⅓ cup dried tart cherries

1 tablespoon melted butter

3 tablespoons brown sugar

¼ teaspoon allspice

Pinch salt

Ice cream, for serving

1. Cut off top ½ inch from each apple; reserve tops. With a melon baller, core through stem ends without breaking through the bottom. (Do not trim bases.)

2. Set the temperature of the air fryer oven to 350ºF (177ºC). Press Start to begin preheating. Combine pecans, cherries, butter, brown sugar, allspice, and a pinch of salt. Stuff mixture into the hollow centers of the apples. Cover with apple tops. Put in the air fryer oven perforated pan, using tongs. Air fry for 20 to 25 minutes, or just until tender.

3. Serve warm with ice cream.

Pineapple and Chocolate Cake

Prep time: 10 minutes | Cook time: 35 to 40 minutes | Serves 4

2 cups flour

4 ounces (113 g) butter, melted

¼ cup sugar

½ pound (227 g) pineapple, chopped

½ cup pineapple juice

1 ounce (28 g) dark chocolate, grated

1 large egg

2 tablespoons skimmed milk

1. Set the temperature of the air fryer oven to 370ºF (188ºC). Press Start to begin preheating.

2. Grease a cake tin with a little oil or butter.

3. In a bowl, combine the butter and flour to create a crumbly consistency.

4. Add the sugar, chopped pineapple, juice, and grated dark chocolate and mix well.

5. In a separate bowl, combine the egg and milk. Add this mixture to the flour mixture and stir well until a soft dough forms.

6. Pour the mixture into the cake tin and transfer to the air fryer oven.

7. Bake for 35 to 40 minutes.

8. Serve immediately.

Pineapple Galette

Prep time: 10 minutes | Cook time: 40 minutes | Serves 2

¼ medium-size pineapple, peeled, cored, and cut crosswise into ¼-inch-thick slices

2 tablespoons dark rum

1 teaspoon vanilla extract

½ teaspoon kosher salt

Finely grated zest of ½ lime

1 store-bought sheet puff pastry, cut into an 8-inch round

3 tablespoons granulated sugar

2 tablespoons unsalted butter, cubed and chilled

Coconut ice cream, for serving

1. Set the temperature of the air fryer oven to 310ºF (154ºC). Press Start to begin preheating.

2. In a small bowl, combine the pineapple slices, rum, vanilla, salt, and lime zest and let stand for at least 10 minutes to allow the pineapple to soak in the rum.

3. Meanwhile, press the puff pastry round into the bottom and up the sides of a round metal cake pan and use the tines of a fork to dock the bottom and sides.

4. Arrange the pineapple slices on the bottom of the pastry in more or less a single layer, then sprinkle with the sugar and dot with the butter. Drizzle with the leftover juices from the bowl. Put the pan in the air fryer oven and bake until the pastry is puffed and golden brown and the pineapple is lightly caramelized on top, about 40 minutes.

5. Transfer the pan to a wire rack to cool for 15 minutes. Unmold the galette from the pan and serve warm with coconut ice cream.

Pumpkin Pudding

Prep time: 10 minutes | Cook time: 15 minutes | Serves 4

3 cups pumpkin purée

3 tablespoons honey

1 tablespoon ginger

1 tablespoon cinnamon

1 teaspoon clove

1 teaspoon nutmeg

1 cup full-fat cream

2 eggs

1 cup sugar

1. Set the temperature of the air fryer oven to 390ºF (199ºC). Press Start to begin preheating.

2. In a bowl, stir all the ingredients together to combine.

3. Grease the inside of a small baking dish.

4. Pour the mixture into the dish and transfer to the air fryer oven. Bake for 15 minutes. Serve warm.

Rich Chocolate Cookie

Prep time: 10 minutes | Cook time: 9 minutes | Serves 4

Nonstick baking spray with flour

3 tablespoons softened butter

$^1/_3$ cup plus 1 tablespoon brown sugar

1 egg yolk

½ cup flour

2 tablespoons ground white chocolate

¼ teaspoon baking soda

½ teaspoon vanilla

¾ cup chocolate chips

1. Set the temperature of the air fryer oven to 350ºF (177ºC). Press Start to begin preheating.

2. In a medium bowl, beat the butter and brown sugar together until fluffy. Stir in the egg yolk.

3. Add the flour, white chocolate, baking soda, and vanilla, and mix well. Stir in the chocolate chips.

4. Line a baking pan with parchment paper. Spray the parchment paper with nonstick baking spray with flour.

5. Spread the batter into the prepared pan, leaving a ½-inch border on all sides.

6. Bake for about 9 minutes or until the cookie is light brown and just barely set.

7. Remove the pan from the air fryer oven and let cool for 10 minutes. Remove the cookie from the pan, remove the parchment paper, and let cool on a wire rack.

8. Serve immediately.

Ricotta Lemon Poppy Seed Cake

Prep time: 15 minutes | Cook time: 55 minutes | Serves 4

Unsalted butter, at room temperature

1 cup almond flour

½ cup sugar

3 large eggs

¼ cup heavy cream

¼ cup full-fat ricotta cheese

¼ cup coconut oil, melted

2 tablespoons poppy seeds

1 teaspoon baking powder

1 teaspoon pure lemon extract

Grated zest and juice of 1 lemon, plus more zest for garnish

1. Set the temperature of the air fryer oven to 325ºF (163ºC). Press Start to begin preheating.

2. Generously butter a round baking pan. Line the bottom of the pan with parchment paper cut to fit.

3. In a large bowl, combine the almond flour, sugar, eggs, cream, ricotta, coconut oil, poppy seeds, baking powder, lemon extract, lemon zest, and lemon juice. Beat with a hand mixer on medium speed until well blended and fluffy.

4. Pour the batter into the prepared pan. Cover the pan tightly with aluminum foil. Set the pan in the air fryer oven and bake for 45 minutes. Remove the foil and bake for 10 to 15 minutes more until a knife (do not use a toothpick) inserted into the center of the cake comes out clean.

5. Let the cake cool in the pan on a wire rack for 10 minutes. Remove the cake from pan and let it cool on the rack for 15 minutes before slicing.

6. Top with additional lemon zest, slice and serve.

Simple Apple Turnovers

Prep time: 10 minutes | Cook time: 10 minutes | Serves 4

1 apple, peeled, quartered, and thinly sliced

½ teaspoons pumpkin pie spice

Juice of ½ lemon

1 tablespoon granulated sugar

Pinch of kosher salt

6 sheets phyllo dough

1. Set the temperature of the air fryer oven to 330ºF (166ºC). Press Start to begin preheating.

2. In a medium bowl, combine the apple, pumpkin pie spice, lemon juice, granulated sugar, and kosher salt.

3. Cut the phyllo dough sheets into 4 equal pieces and place individual tablespoons of apple filling in the center of each piece, then fold in both sides and roll from front to back.

4. Spray the air fryer oven perforated pan with nonstick cooking spray, then place the turnovers in the perforated pan and bake for 10 minutes or until golden brown.

5. Remove the turnovers from the air fryer oven and allow to cool on a wire rack for 10 minutes before serving.

Simple Pineapple Sticks

Prep time: 5 minutes | Cook time: 10 minutes | Serves 4

½ fresh pineapple, cut into sticks

¼ cup desiccated coconut

1. Set the temperature of the air fryer oven to 400ºF (204ºC). Press Start to begin preheating.

2. Coat the pineapple sticks in the desiccated coconut and put each one in the air fryer oven perforated pan.

3. Air fry for 10 minutes.

4. Serve immediately

Spice Cookies

Prep time: 15 minutes | Cook time: 12 minutes | Serves 4

4 tablespoons (½ stick) unsalted butter, at room temperature

2 tablespoons agave nectar

1 large egg

2 tablespoons water

2½ cups almond flour

½ cup sugar

2 teaspoons ground ginger

1 teaspoon ground cinnamon

½ teaspoon freshly grated nutmeg

1 teaspoon baking soda

¼ teaspoon kosher salt

1. Set the temperature of the air fryer oven to 325ºF (163ºC). Press Start to begin preheating.

2. Line the bottom of the air fryer oven perforated pan with parchment paper cut to fit.

3. In a large bowl using a hand mixer, beat together the butter, agave, egg, and water on medium speed until fluffy.

4. Add the almond flour, sugar, ginger, cinnamon, nutmeg, baking soda, and salt. Beat on low speed until well combined.

5. Roll the dough into 2-tablespoon balls and arrange them on the parchment paper in the perforated pan. Bake for 12 minutes, or until the tops of cookies are lightly browned.

6. Transfer to a wire rack and let cool completely.

7. Serve immediately

Air Fried Baby Back Ribs

Prep time: 5 minutes | Cook time: 30 minutes | Serves 2

2 teaspoons red pepper flakes

¾ ground ginger

3 cloves minced garlic

Salt and ground black pepper, to taste

2 baby back ribs

1. Set the temperature of the air fryer oven to 350ºF (177ºC). Press Start to begin preheating.

2. Combine the red pepper flakes, ginger, garlic, salt and pepper in a bowl, making sure to mix well. Massage the mixture into the baby back ribs.

3. Air fry the ribs in the air fryer oven for 30 minutes.

4. Take care when taking the rubs out of the air fryer oven. Put them on a serving dish and serve.

Air Fried Beef Ribs

Prep time: 20 minutes | Cook time: 8 minutes | Serves 4

1 pound (454 g) meaty beef ribs, rinsed and drained

3 tablespoons apple cider vinegar

1 cup coriander, finely chopped

1 tablespoon fresh basil leaves, chopped

2 garlic cloves, finely chopped

1 chipotle powder

1 teaspoon fennel seeds

1 teaspoon hot paprika

Kosher salt and black pepper, to taste

½ cup vegetable oil

1. Coat the ribs with the remaining ingredients and refrigerate for at least 3 hours.

2. Set the temperature of the air fryer oven to 360ºF (182ºC). Press Start to begin preheating.

3. Separate the ribs from the marinade and put them on a grill pan. Air fry for 8 minutes.

4. Pour the remaining marinade over the ribs before serving.

Air Fried Lamb Ribs

Prep time: 5 minutes | Cook time: 18 minutes | Serves 4

2 tablespoons mustard

1 pound (454 g) lamb ribs

1 teaspoon rosemary, chopped

Salt and ground black pepper, to taste

¼ cup mint leaves, chopped

1 cup Green yogurt

1. Set the temperature of the air fryer oven to 350ºF (177ºC). Press Start to begin preheating.

2. Use a brush to apply the mustard to the lamb ribs, and season with rosemary, salt, and pepper.

3. Air fry the ribs in the air fryer oven for 18 minutes.

4. Meanwhile, combine the mint leaves and yogurt in a bowl.

5. Remove the lamb ribs from the air fryer oven when cooked and serve with the mint yogurt.

Air Fried London Broil

Prep time: 15 minutes | Cook time: 25 minutes | Serves 8

2 pounds (907 g) London broil

3 large garlic cloves, minced

3 tablespoons balsamic vinegar

3 tablespoons whole-grain mustard

2 tablespoons olive oil

Sea salt and ground black pepper, to taste

½ teaspoons dried hot red pepper flakes

1. Wash and dry the London broil. Score its sides with a knife.

2. Mix the remaining ingredients. Rub this mixture into the broil, coating it well. Allow to marinate for a minimum of 3 hours.

3. Set the temperature of the air fryer oven to 400ºF (204ºC). Press Start to begin preheating.

4. Air fry the meat for 15 minutes. Turn it over and air fry for an additional 10 minutes before serving.

Air Fried Ribeye Steak

Prep time: 5 minutes | Cook time: 15 minutes | Serves 1

1 (1-pound / 454-g) ribeye steak

Salt and ground black pepper, to taste

1 tablespoon peanut oil

½ tablespoon butter

½ teaspoon thyme, chopped

1. Set the temperature of the air fryer oven to 400ºF (204ºC). Press Start to begin preheating.

2. Season the steaks with salt and pepper.

3. Grease a skillet with peanut oil. Sear the steak over medium heat for 2 minutes.

4. Turn over the steak and place in the air fryer oven for 6 minutes.

5. Take out the steak from the air fryer oven and place it back on the stove top on low heat to keep warm.

6. Toss in the butter and thyme and air fry for 3 minutes.

7. Rest for 5 minutes and serve.

Avocado Buttered Flank Steak

Prep time: 5 minutes | Cook time: 12 minutes | Serves 1

1 flank steak

Salt and ground black pepper, to taste

2 avocados

2 tablespoons butter, melted

½ cup chimichurri sauce

1. Rub the flank steak with salt and pepper to taste and leave to sit for 20 minutes.

2. Set the temperature of the air fryer oven to 400ºF (204ºC) and place a rack inside.

3. Halve the avocados and take out the pits. Spoon the flesh into a bowl and mash with a fork. Mix in the melted butter and chimichurri sauce, making sure everything is well combined.

4. Put the steak in the air fryer oven and air fry for 6 minutes. Flip over and allow to air fry for another 6 minutes.

5. Serve the steak with the avocado butter.

Bacon and Pear Stuffed Pork Chops

Prep time: 20 minutes | Cook time: 24 minutes | Serves 3

4 slices bacon, chopped

1 tablespoon butter

½ cup finely diced onion

⅓ cup chicken stock

1½ cups seasoned stuffing cubes

1 egg, beaten

½ teaspoon dried thyme

½ teaspoon salt

⅛ teaspoon freshly ground black pepper

1 pear, finely diced

⅓ cup crumbled blue cheese

3 boneless center-cut pork chops (2-inch thick)

Olive oil, for greasing

Salt and freshly ground black pepper, to taste

1. Set the temperature of the air fryer oven to 400ºF (204ºC). Press Start to begin preheating.

2. Put the bacon into the air fryer oven perforated pan and air fry for 6 minutes, stirring halfway through the cooking time. Remove the bacon and set it aside on a

paper towel. Pour out the grease from the bottom of the air fryer oven.

3. To make the stuffing, melt the butter in a medium saucepan over medium heat on the stovetop. Add the onion and sauté for a few minutes until it starts to soften. Add the chicken stock and simmer for 1 minute. Remove the pan from the heat and add the stuffing cubes. Stir until the stock has been absorbed. Add the egg, dried thyme, salt and freshly ground black pepper, and stir until combined. Fold in the diced pear and crumbled blue cheese.

4. Put the pork chops on a cutting board. Using the palm of the hand to hold the chop flat and steady, slice into the side of the pork chop to make a pocket in the center of the chop. Leave about an inch of chop uncut and make sure you don't cut all the way through the pork chop. Brush both sides of the pork chops with olive oil and season with salt and freshly ground black pepper. Stuff each pork chop with a third of the stuffing, packing the stuffing tightly inside the pocket.

5. Set the temperature of the air fryer oven to 360ºF (182ºC). Press Start to begin preheating.

6. Spray or brush the sides of the air fryer oven perforated pan with oil. Put the pork chops in the perforated pan

with the open, stuffed edge of the pork chop facing the outside edges of the perforated pan.

7. Air fry the pork chops for 18 minutes, turning the pork chops over halfway through the cooking time. When the chops are done, let them rest for 5 minutes and then transfer to a serving platter.

Bacon Wrapped Pork with Apple Gravy

Prep time: 10 minutes | Cook time: 25 minutes | Serves 4

Pork:

1 tablespoons Dijon mustard

1 pork tenderloin

3 strips bacon

Apple Gravy:

3 tablespoons ghee, divided

1 shallot, chopped

2 apples

1 tablespoon almond flour

1 cup vegetable broth

½ teaspoon Dijon mustard

1. Set the temperature of the air fryer oven to 360ºF (182ºC). Press Start to begin preheating.
2. Spread Dijon mustard all over tenderloin and wrap meat with strips of bacon.
3. Put into air fryer oven and air fry for 12 minutes. Use a meat thermometer to check for doneness.
4. To make sauce, heat 1 tablespoon of ghee in a pan and add shallots. Cook for 1 minute.
5. Then add apples, cooking for 4 minutes until softened.

6. Add flour and 2 tablespoons of ghee to make a roux. Add broth and mustard, stirring well to combine.

7. When sauce starts to bubble, add 1 cup of sautéed apples, cooking until sauce thickens.

8. Once pork tenderloin is cooked, allow to sit 8 minutes to rest before slicing.

9. Serve topped with apple gravy.

Barbecue Pork Ribs

Prep time: 5 minutes | Cook time: 30 minutes | Serves 4

1 tablespoon barbecue dry rub

1 teaspoon mustard

1 tablespoon apple cider vinegar

1 teaspoon sesame oil

1 pound (454 g) pork ribs, chopped

1. Combine the dry rub, mustard, apple cider vinegar, and sesame oil, then coat the ribs with this mixture. Refrigerate the ribs for 20 minutes.

2. Set the temperature of the air fryer oven to 360ºF (182ºC). Press Start to begin preheating.

3. When the ribs are ready, place them in the air fryer oven and air fry for 15 minutes. Flip them and air fry on the other side for a further 15 minutes.

4. Serve immediately.

BBQ Pork Steaks

Prep time: 5 minutes | Cook time: 15 minutes | Serves 4

4 pork steaks

1 tablespoon Cajun seasoning

2 tablespoons BBQ sauce

1 tablespoon vinegar

1 teaspoon soy sauce

½ cup brown sugar

½ cup ketchup

1. Set the temperature of the air fryer oven to 290ºF (143ºC). Press Start to begin preheating.

2. Sprinkle pork steaks with Cajun seasoning.

3. Combine remaining ingredients and brush onto steaks.

4. Add coated steaks to air fryer oven. Air fry 15 minutes until just browned.

5. Serve immediately.

Beef and Cheddar Burgers

Prep time: 20 minutes | Cook time: 25 minutes | Serves 4

1 tablespoon olive oil

1 onion, sliced into rings

1 teaspoon garlic, minced or puréed

1 teaspoon mustard

1 teaspoon basil

1 teaspoon mixed herbs

Salt and ground black pepper, to taste

1 teaspoon tomato, puréed

4 buns

1 ounce (28 g) Cheddar cheese

10.5 ounces (298 g) beef, minced

Salad leaves

1. Set the temperature of the air fryer oven to 390ºF (199ºC). Press Start to begin preheating.

2. Grease the air fryer oven with olive oil and allow it to warm up.

3. Put the diced onion in the air fryer oven and air fry until they turn golden brown.

4. Mix the garlic, mustard, basil, herbs, salt, and pepper, and air fry for 25 minutes.

5. Lay 2 to 3 onion rings and puréed tomato on two of the buns. Put one slice of cheese and the layer of beef on top. Top with salad leaves and any other condiments you desire before closing off the sandwich with the other buns.

6. Serve immediately.

Beef and Pork Sausage Meatloaf

Prep time: 20 minutes | Cook time: 25 minutes | Serves 4

¾ pound (340 g) ground chuck

4 ounces (113 g) ground pork sausage

1 cup shallots, finely chopped

2 eggs, well beaten

3 tablespoons plain milk

1 tablespoon oyster sauce

1 teaspoon porcini mushrooms

½ teaspoon cumin powder

1 teaspoon garlic paste

1 tablespoon fresh parsley

Salt and crushed red pepper flakes, to taste

1 cup crushed saltines

Cooking spray

1. Set the temperature of the air fryer oven to 360ºF (182ºC). Press Start to begin preheating. Spritz a baking dish with cooking spray.

2. Mix all the ingredients in a large bowl, combining everything well.

3. Transfer to the baking dish and bake in the air fryer oven for 25 minutes.

4. Serve hot.

Beef and Spinach Rolls

Prep time: 10 minutes | Cook time: 14 minutes | Serves 2

3 teaspoons pesto

2 pounds (907 g) beef flank steak

6 slices provolone cheese

3 ounces (85 g) roasted red bell peppers

¾ cup baby spinach

1 teaspoon sea salt

1 teaspoon black pepper

1. Set the temperature of the air fryer oven to 400ºF (204ºC). Press Start to begin preheating.

2. Spoon equal amounts of the pesto onto each flank steak and spread it across evenly.

3. Put the cheese, roasted red peppers and spinach on top of the meat, about three-quarters of the way down.

4. Roll the steak up, holding it in place with toothpicks. Sprinkle with the sea salt and pepper.

5. Put inside the air fryer oven and air fry for 14 minutes, turning halfway through the cooking time.

6. Allow the beef to rest for 10 minutes before slicing up and serving.

Beef and Vegetable Cubes

Prep time: 15 minutes | Cook time: 17 minutes | Serves 4

2 tablespoons olive oil

1 tablespoon apple cider vinegar

1 teaspoon fine sea salt

½ teaspoons ground black pepper

1 teaspoon shallot powder

¾ teaspoon smoked cayenne pepper

½ teaspoons garlic powder

¼ teaspoon ground cumin

1 pound (454 g) top round steak, cut into cubes

4 ounces (113 g) broccoli, cut into florets

4 ounces (113 g) mushrooms, sliced

1 teaspoon dried basil

1 teaspoon celery seeds

1. Massage the olive oil, vinegar, salt, black pepper, shallot powder, cayenne pepper, garlic powder, and cumin into the cubed steak, ensuring to coat each piece evenly.

2. Allow to marinate for a minimum of 3 hours.

3. Set the temperature of the air fryer oven to 365ºF (185ºC). Press Start to begin preheating.

4. Put the beef cubes in the air fryer oven perforated pan and air fry for 12 minutes.

5. When the steak is cooked through, place it in a bowl.

6. Wipe the grease from the perforated pan and pour in the vegetables. Season them with basil and celery seeds.

7. Increase the temperature of the air fryer oven to 400ºF (204ºC) and air fry for 5 to 6 minutes. When the vegetables are hot, serve them with the steak.

Beef Cheeseburger Egg Rolls

Prep time: 15 minutes | Cook time: 8 minutes | Makes 6 egg rolls

8 ounces (227 g) raw lean ground beef

½ cup chopped onion

½ cup chopped bell pepper

¼ teaspoon onion powder

¼ teaspoon garlic powder

3 tablespoons cream cheese

1 tablespoon yellow mustard

3 tablespoons shredded Cheddar cheese

6 chopped dill pickle chips

6 egg roll wrappers

1. Set the temperature of the air fryer oven to 392ºF (200ºC). Press Start to begin preheating.

2. In a skillet, add the beef, onion, bell pepper, onion powder, and garlic powder. Stir and crumble beef until fully cooked, and vegetables are soft.

3. Take skillet off the heat and add cream cheese, mustard, and Cheddar cheese, stirring until melted.

4. Pour beef mixture into a bowl and fold in pickles.

5. Lay out egg wrappers and divide the beef mixture into each one. Moisten egg roll wrapper edges with water. Fold sides to the middle and seal with water.

6. Repeat with all other egg rolls.

7. Put rolls into air fryer oven, one batch at a time. Air fry for 8 minutes.

8. Serve immediately.

Beef Chuck Cheeseburgers

Prep time: 10 minutes | Cook time: 15 minutes | Serves 4

¾ pound (340 g) ground beef chuck

1 envelope onion soup mix

Kosher salt and freshly ground black pepper, to taste

1 teaspoon paprika

4 slices Monterey Jack cheese

4 ciabatta rolls

1. In a bowl, stir together the ground chuck, onion soup mix, salt, black pepper, and paprika to combine well.

2. Set the temperature of the air fryer oven to 385ºF (196ºC). Press Start to begin preheating.

3. Take four equal portions of the mixture and mold each one into a patty. Transfer to the air fryer oven and air fry for 10 minutes.

4. Put the slices of cheese on the top of the burgers.

5. Air fry for another minute before serving on ciabatta rolls.

Beef Chuck with Brussels Sprouts

Prep time: 20 minutes | Cook time: 15 minutes | Serves 4

1 pound (454 g) beef chuck shoulder steak

2 tablespoons vegetable oil

1 tablespoon red wine vinegar

1 teaspoon fine sea salt

½ teaspoon ground black pepper

1 teaspoon smoked paprika

1 teaspoon onion powder

½ teaspoon garlic powder

½ pound (227 g) Brussels sprouts, cleaned and halved

½ teaspoon fennel seeds

1 teaspoon dried basil

1 teaspoon dried sage

1. Massage the beef with the vegetable oil, wine vinegar, salt, black pepper, paprika, onion powder, and garlic powder, coating it well.

2. Allow to marinate for a minimum of 3 hours.

3. Set the temperature of the air fryer oven to 390ºF (199ºC). Press Start to begin preheating.

4. Remove the beef from the marinade and put in the preheated air fryer oven. Air fry for 10 minutes. Flip the beef halfway through.

5. Put the prepared Brussels sprouts in the air fryer oven along with the fennel seeds, basil, and sage.

6. Lower the heat to 380ºF (193ºC) and air fry everything for another 5 minutes.

7. Give them a good stir. Air fry for an additional 10 minutes.

8. Serve immediately.

Beef Egg Rolls

Prep time: 15 minutes | Cook time: 12 minutes | Makes 8 egg rolls

½ chopped onion

2 garlic cloves, chopped

½ packet taco seasoning

Salt and ground black pepper, to taste

1 pound (454 g) lean ground beef

½ can cilantro lime rotel

16 egg roll wrappers

1 cup shredded Mexican cheese

1 tablespoon olive oil

1 teaspoon cilantro

1. Set the temperature of the air fryer oven to 400ºF (205ºC). Press Start to begin preheating.

2. Add onions and garlic to a skillet, cooking until fragrant. Then add taco seasoning, pepper, salt, and beef, cooking until beef is broke up into tiny pieces and cooked thoroughly.

3. Add rotel and stir well.

4. Lay out egg wrappers and brush with a touch of water to soften a bit.

5. Load wrappers with beef filling and add cheese to each.

6. Fold diagonally to close and use water to secure edges.

7. Brush filled egg wrappers with olive oil and add to the air fryer oven.

8. Air fry 8 minutes, flip, and air fry for another 4 minutes.

9. Serve sprinkled with cilantro.

Beef Loin with Thyme and Parsley

Prep time: 5 minutes | Cook time: 15 minutes | Serves 4

1 tablespoon butter, melted

¼ dried thyme

1 teaspoon garlic salt

¼ teaspoon dried parsley

1 pound (454 g) beef loin

1. In a bowl, combine the melted butter, thyme, garlic salt, and parsley.

2. Cut the beef loin into slices and generously apply the seasoned butter using a brush.

3. Set the temperature of the air fryer oven to 400ºF (204ºC) and place a rack inside.

4. Air fry the beef on the rack for 15 minutes.

5. Take care when removing it and serve hot.

Beef Steak Fingers

Prep time: 5 minutes | Cook time: 8 minutes | Serves 4

4 small beef cube steaks

Salt and ground black pepper, to taste

½ cup flour

Cooking spray

1. Set the temperature of the air fryer oven to 390ºF (199ºC). Press Start to begin preheating.

2. Cut cube steaks into 1-inch-wide strips.

3. Sprinkle lightly with salt and pepper to taste.

4. Roll in flour to coat all sides.

5. Spritz air fryer oven perforated pan with cooking spray.

6. Put steak strips in air fryer oven perforated pan in a single layer. Spritz top of steak strips with oil or cooking spray.

7. Air fry for 4 minutes, turn strips over, and spritz with cooking spray.

8. Air fry 4 more minutes and test with fork for doneness. Steak fingers should be crispy outside with no red juices inside.

9. Repeat steps 5 through 7 to air fry remaining strips.

10. Serve immediately.

Carne Asada Tacos

Prep time: 5 minutes | Cook time: 14 minutes | Serves 4

$^1/_3$ cup olive oil

1½ pounds (680 g) flank steak

Salt and freshly ground black pepper, to taste

$^1/_3$ cup freshly squeezed lime juice

½ cup chopped fresh cilantro

4 teaspoons minced garlic

1 teaspoon ground cumin

1 teaspoon chili powder

1. Brush the air fryer oven perforated pan with olive oil.

2. Put the flank steak in a large mixing bowl. Season with salt and pepper.

3. Add the lime juice, cilantro, garlic, cumin, and chili powder and toss to coat the steak.

4. For the best flavor, let the steak marinate in the refrigerator for about 1 hour.

5. Set the temperature of the air fryer oven to 400ºF (204ºC)

6. Put the steak in the air fryer oven perforated pan. Air fry for 7 minutes. Flip the steak. Air fry for 7 minutes more

or until an internal temperature reaches at least 145ºF (63ºC).

7. Let the steak rest for about 5 minutes, then cut into strips to serve.

Char Siew

Prep time: 10 minutes | Cook time: 20 minutes | Serves 4 to 6

1 strip of pork shoulder butt with a good amount of fat marbling

Olive oil, for brushing the pan

Marinade:

1 teaspoon sesame oil

4 tablespoons raw honey

1 teaspoon low-sodium dark soy sauce

1 teaspoon light soy sauce

1 tablespoon rose wine

2 tablespoons Hoisin sauce

1. Combine the marinade ingredients together in a Ziploc bag. Put pork in bag, making sure all sections of pork strip are engulfed in the marinade. Chill for at least 3 hours.

2. Take out the strip 30 minutes before planning to roast and set the temperature of the air fryer oven to 350ºF (177ºC). Press Start to begin preheating.

3. Put foil on small pan and brush with olive oil. Put marinated pork strip onto prepared pan.

4. Roast in the air fryer oven for 20 minutes.

5. Glaze with marinade every 5 to 10 minutes.

6. Remove strip and leave to cool a few minutes before slicing.

7. Serve immediately.

Cheddar Bacon Burst with Spinach

Prep time: 5 minutes | Cook time: 60 minutes | Serves 8

30 slices bacon

1 tablespoon Chipotle seasoning

2 teaspoons Italian seasoning

2½ cups Cheddar cheese

4 cups raw spinach

1. Set the temperature of the air fryer oven to 375ºF (191ºC). Press Start to begin preheating.

2. Weave the bacon into 15 vertical pieces and 12 horizontal pieces. Cut the extra 3 in half to fill in the rest, horizontally.

3. Season the bacon with Chipotle seasoning and Italian seasoning.

4. Add the cheese to the bacon.

5. Add the spinach and press down to compress.

6. Tightly roll up the woven bacon.

7. Line a baking sheet with kitchen foil and add plenty of salt to it.

8. Put the bacon on top of a cooling rack and put that on top of the baking sheet.

9. Bake for 60 minutes.

10. Let cool for 15 minutes before slicing and serve.

Cheese Crusted Chops

Prep time: 10 minutes | Cook time: 12 minutes | Serves 4 to 6

¼ teaspoon pepper

½ teaspoons salt

4 to 6 thick boneless pork chops

1 cup pork rind crumbs

¼ teaspoon chili powder

½ teaspoons onion powder

1 teaspoon smoked paprika

2 beaten eggs

3 tablespoons grated Parmesan cheese

Cooking spray

1. Set the temperature of the air fryer oven to 400ºF (205ºC). Press Start to begin preheating.

2. Rub the pepper and salt on both sides of pork chops.

3. In a food processor, pulse pork rinds into crumbs. Mix crumbs with chili powder, onion powder, and paprika in a bowl.

4. Beat eggs in another bowl.

5. Dip pork chops into eggs then into pork rind crumb mixture.

6. Spritz the air fryer oven with cooking spray and add pork chops to the perforated pan.

7. Air fry for 12 minutes.

8. Serve garnished with the Parmesan cheese.

Cheesy Beef Meatballs

Prep time: 5 minutes | Cook time: 18 minutes | Serves 6

1 pound (454 g) ground beef

½ cup grated Parmesan cheese

1 tablespoon minced garlic

½ cup Mozzarella cheese

1 teaspoon freshly ground pepper

1. Set the temperature of the air fryer oven to 400ºF (204ºC). Press Start to begin preheating.

2. In a bowl, mix all the ingredients together.

3. Roll the meat mixture into 5 generous meatballs.

4. Air fry inside the air fryer oven at 165ºF (74ºC) for about 18 minutes.

5. Serve immediately.

Chicken Fried Steak

Prep time: 15 minutes | Cook time: 10 minutes | Serves 4

½ cup flour

2 teaspoons salt, divided

Freshly ground black pepper, to taste

¼ teaspoon garlic powder

1 cup buttermilk

1 cup fine bread crumbs

4 (6-ounce / 170-g) tenderized top round steaks, ½-inch thick

Vegetable or canola oil

For the Gravy:

2 tablespoons butter or bacon drippings

¼ onion, minced

1 clove garlic, smashed

¼ teaspoon dried thyme

3 tablespoons flour

1 cup milk

Salt and freshly ground black pepper, to taste

Dashes of Worcestershire sauce

1. Set up a dredging station. Combine the flour, 1 teaspoon of salt, black pepper and garlic powder in a shallow

bowl. Pour the buttermilk into a second shallow bowl. Finally, put the bread crumbs and 1 teaspoon of salt in a third shallow bowl.

2. Dip the tenderized steaks into the flour, then the buttermilk, and then the bread crumb mixture, pressing the crumbs onto the steak. Put them on a baking sheet and spray both sides generously with vegetable or canola oil.

3. Set the temperature of the air fryer oven to 400ºF (204ºC). Press Start to begin preheating.

4. Transfer the steaks to the air fryer oven perforated pan, two at a time, and air fry for 10 minutes, flipping the steaks over halfway through the cooking time.

5. While the steaks are cooking, make the gravy. Melt the butter in a small saucepan over medium heat on the stovetop. Add the onion, garlic and thyme and cook for five minutes, until the onion is soft and just starting to brown. Stir in the flour and cook for another five minutes, stirring regularly, until the mixture starts to brown. Whisk in the milk and bring the mixture to a boil to thicken. Season to taste with salt, lots of freshly ground black pepper, and a few dashes of Worcestershire sauce.

6. Pour the gravy over the chicken fried steaks and serve.

Citrus Pork Loin Roast

Prep time: 10 minutes | Cook time: 45 minutes | Serves 8

1 tablespoon lime juice

1 tablespoon orange marmalade

1 teaspoon coarse brown mustard

1 teaspoon curry powder

1 teaspoon dried lemongrass

2 pound (907 g) boneless pork loin roast

Salt and ground black pepper, to taste

Cooking spray

1. Set the temperature of the air fryer oven to 360ºF (182ºC). Press Start to begin preheating.

2. Mix the lime juice, marmalade, mustard, curry powder, and lemongrass.

3. Rub mixture all over the surface of the pork loin. Season with salt and pepper.

4. Spray air fryer oven perforated pan with cooking spray and place pork roast diagonally in the perforated pan.

5. Air fry for approximately 45 minutes, until the internal temperature reaches at least 145ºF (63ºC).

6. Wrap roast in foil and let rest for 10 minutes before slicing.

7. Serve immediately.

Classic Spring Rolls

Prep time: 10 minutes | Cook time: 8 minutes | Serves 20

$^1/_3$ cup noodles

1 cup ground beef

1 teaspoon soy sauce

1 cup fresh mix vegetables

3 garlic cloves, minced

1 small onion, diced

1 tablespoon sesame oil

1 packet spring roll sheets

2 tablespoons cold water

1. Cook the noodle in enough hot water to soften them up, drain them and snip them to make them shorter.

2. In a frying pan over medium heat, cook the beef, soy sauce, mixed vegetables, garlic, and onion in sesame oil until the beef is cooked through. Take the pan off the heat and throw in the noodles. Mix well to incorporate everything.

3. Unroll a spring roll sheet and lay it flat. Scatter the filling diagonally across it and roll it up, brushing the edges

lightly with water to act as an adhesive. Repeat until you have used up all the sheets and the filling.

4. Set the temperature of the air fryer oven to 350ºF (177ºC). Press Start to begin preheating.

5. Coat each spring roll with a light brushing of oil and transfer to the air fryer oven.

6. Air fry for 8 minutes and serve hot.

CPSIA information can be obtained
at www.ICGtesting.com
Printed in the USA
BVHW012316070722
641302BV00027B/392